DEDICATION

To the well being of our patients who have questions and look to us and our colleagues for answers. May our combined knowledge and skill help guide you through the surgical experience.

We thank you for trusting in us.

and

To Mignonne and "Babe" Mailhot, my parents, who instilled in me the strength and perseverance to achieve my personal and professional goals.

CLAIRE MAILHOT

To my husband, "Bru," for his love, and to my parents, Ernie and Chris Alves, for their encouragement.

MELINDA ALVES BRUBAKER

To my parents, Bob and Marie Garratt, for their gifts of love and laughter and for believing in me.

LINDA GARRATT SLEZAK

AUTHORS

CLAIRE MAILHOT, RN, MS, EdD, FAAN
Service Line Administrator
UCSF Stanford Health Care

MELINDA BRUBAKER, RN, BSN
Health Care Consultant

LINDA GARRATT SLEZAK, RN, MS, FAAN
Health Care Surgical Consultant

CONTRIBUTING AUTHORS

LAURA ADAMS, BS
Administrative Director
Bone Marrow and Stem Cell Transplantation
Duke University Health System

TERRI HOMER, MD
Clinical Assistant Professor
Department of Anesthesia
Stanford University School of Medicine

ROSEMARY MANN, RN, CNM, JD, PhD
Assistant Professor
San Jose State University
School of Nursing

SURGERY

A Patient's Guide from Diagnosis to Recovery

Claire Mailhot

Melinda Brubaker

Linda Garratt Slezak

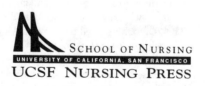

SCHOOL OF NURSING
UNIVERSITY OF CALIFORNIA, SAN FRANCISCO
UCSF NURSING PRESS

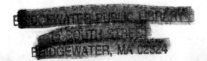

Senior Publications Coordinator: Kathleen McClung
Design/Production: Patricia Walsh Design
Editor: Lisa Carlson
Proofreader: Cheryl Cohen

For information, contact:

UCSF Nursing Press
School of Nursing
University of California, San Francisco
521 Parnassus Avenue, Room N535C
San Francisco, CA 94143-0608 U.S.A.
Phone: (415)476-4992
Fax: (415)476-6042
Internet: http://nurseweb.ucsf.edu/www/books.htm

ISBN: 0-943671-19-1

First Printing, 1999
Printed in U.S.A.

Disclaimer

This book has been written to guide patients and family members diagnosed with an illness or those who have had an accident that will result in
the need for surgery. This is a tool intended to help in talking with health
care professionals and to help you to prepare for surgery.

Each person's situation and needs are different. This book may not
answer all your specific, disease-related questions, and as such does not
replace the communication you must establish with your physician or nursing
staff. It is intended as a guide for dialogue and provides ways to capture information and suggestions or ways to maintain your well-being while in the hospital or during post surgical procedure.

Claire Mailhot

Claire B. Mailhot, RN, MS, EdD, FAAN, is Director of Surgical Program Developments at Stanford University Hospital and a nationally recognized authority on operating room management. Her 25-year career encompasses a wide variety of both clinical and administrative positions, giving her a broad perspective on all aspects of the surgical experience.

Claire is Editor-in-Chief of *Advanced Training for Operating Room Clinical Specialties* (Medcom, Inc., 1992-1994), an award-winning series of learning modules for surgical nurses. She is also Editor-in-Chief of *Management Training for Today's OR* (Medcom, Inc., in press). Additionally, she has published numerous articles on operating room management in leading professional journals.

A frequent speaker at national industry forums, Claire also serves on the advisory boards of numerous health care organizations and publications. She has additionally served as a consultant to international health care organizations on various aspects of operating room management.

Claire is the recipient of several prestigious industry awards. In 1994, she was appointed a Fellow in the American Academy of Nursing. She was also awarded the Certificate of Excellence from the Health Services Communication Association (HESCA) in 1993.

Claire received a Bachelor of Science degree in Nursing from California State University, San Francisco; a Masters of Science degree in Nursing Administration from the University of California, San Francisco; and a Doctor of Education degree from the University of San Francisco. She also completed a Post Doctoral Fellowship in Management Development at Stanford University.

Melinda (Alves) Brubaker

Melinda (Alves) Brubaker, RN, BSN, began her nursing career in a large academic medical center as a staff nurse on a postoperative cardiovascular surgery unit. She subsequently transferred to the Emergency Department where she held several positions, including staff nurse, nurse educator, paramedic educator, and nurse administrator. Currently she does health care consulting and works part-time for the University of Southern Maine's Edmund S. Muskie School of Public Service, Institute for Public Sector Innovation. At "Muskie" she is involved in an innovative collaborative partnership between academia and government agencies that focuses on teaching, research, and public service.

Linda Garratt Slezak

Linda Slezak, RN, MS, FAAN, is a Surgical Services Executive Consultant for APM Incorporated. In this role she works with hospitals around the country to improve patient flow and efficiency of surgical services. She is past Director of Surgical Services and Assistant Director of Nursing at Stanford University Hospital, with management responsibility for the 20-suite main operating room and the 10-suite Ambulatory Surgery Center. Since joining Stanford in 1973, Linda served in a variety of both clinical and administrative positions, winning numerous laurels for her achievements. Most recently, as testimony to her leadership and expertise, Stanford's operating room region was rated one of the nations' best in a national benchmarking study conducted in 1995 by the University Hospital Consortium (UHC).

Linda is Associate Editor of *Advanced Training for Operating Room Clinical Specialties* (Medcom, Inc., 1992-1994), a widely utilized series of learning modules for surgical nurses. She is also Associate Editor of *Management Training for Today's OR* (Medcom, Inc., in press). She currently serves on the Nursing Advisory Board for Medcom, Inc. and is on the Editorial Board of *OR Report*. She has published numerous articles in professional journals.

Linda is a frequent lecturer before leading industry groups and has participated on several national committees addressing key operating room issues. She has also provided consultation to university teaching hospitals in Russia, Japan, and Israel.

Linda's expertise is marked by the numerous industry awards she has received and her most recent appointment as a Fellow in the American Academy of Nursing.

Linda received a Bachelor of Science degree in Nursing from California State University, San Francisco and a Master of Science degree in Nursing Administration from the University of California, San Francisco.

Laura Adams

Laura L. Adams, BS, is the Administrative Director for the adult and pediatric Bone Marrow and Stem Cell Transplant Programs at Duke University Health System. Ms. Adams has responsibility for developing and implementing strategies which will enhance Duke's position as a leader in transplantation, and for successfully integrating managed care into the program. Ms. Adams also serves as a managed care consultant for other academic centers.

Laura has over 14 years' experience in managed health care. Prior to coming to Duke in 1998, she was at Stanford Health Services/Lucile Salter Packard Children's Hospital at Stanford for seven years as the Senior Manager of Specialty Contracting. In this capacity Laura increased the number of transplant managed care contracts from 20 to over 150, and managed over $65 million in annual revenue for the medical center. Laura has also worked for Travelers Insurance Company and Healthcare Management Consultants. She received her Bachelor's of Science from Old Dominion University in Virginia.

Terri Homer

Terri Homer, M.D., is a Board Certified anesthesiologist in full-time practice in Palo Alto, California. She received her M.D. at Northwestern Medical School and completed her anesthesia residency and fellowship at Stanford University Medical School in 1983. She is a professional employee of the Associated Anesthesiologists Medical Group and is on the active medical staff at UCSF Stanford Health Care, Lucile Salter Packard Children's Hospital at Stanford, and many outpatient surgery centers in the community. In addition to this work, she has developed an office anesthesia practice which involves sedating children and adults in medical, dental, and oral surgery offices. This is a relatively new frontier, and Terri lectures about this work at national meetings. She is an active member of the American Society of Office Based Anesthesia. In addition to her usual work, Terri has traveled to developing countries with Interplast since 1982. She has made over 18 trips to work as a volunteer anesthesiologist to care for children with burns and other congenital deformities needing corrective surgery. She also serves on the Board of Directors of Interplast, headquartered in Mountain View, California.

Rosemary J. Mann

Rosemary J. Mann, R.N., C.N.M., J.D., Ph.D. is currently Assistant Professor and Undergraduate Coordinator at the San Jose State University School of Nursing. She completed a B.S.N. at Western Reserve University, an M.S.N. and Certificate of Nurse-Midwifery at Columbia University, a J.D. at the University of San Francisco, and a Ph.D. at the University of California, San Francisco. She currently practices nurse-midwifery on a per diem basis at several community clinics and offers professional consultation on legal and ethical issues related to advance practice nursing. She is President of the California Nurse-Midwives Association.

ACKNOWLEDGEMENTS

Jeanne DeJoseph, Ph.D., C.N.M., F.A.A.N., Associate Professor and Co-Director, Nurse Midwifery Education, UCSF School of Nursing

Suzanne Dibble, DNSc, R.N., Associate Adjunct Professor, Institute of Health and Aging, Department of Physiological Nursing, UCSF School of Nursing

Camran Nezhat, M.D., Clinical Professor, Department of Gynecology and Obstetrics

Linda Cook, R.N., Assistant Nurse Manager, General Surgery and Transplant

Patricia Daniels, Director Patient Admitting Services, Stanford University Hospital

Carol Oakes, R.N., M.S., Nursing Supervisor

Pam McFarlin, R.N., M.S., Program Manager, Home Care, UCSF Stanford Health Care

Lisa Merenback, M.H.S.A., Assistant Director, Health Plan Services, UCSF Stanford Health Care

Diana Davis, Administrative Assistant

Sue Anselowitz, R.N., Post Anesthesia Care Nurse

Cecilia Montavo, Vice President, Medicare and Choice Division, Brown and Toland, Inc.

Deb Walt, Marketing Communications Consultant

Sara White, M.S., Stanford Pharmacy Director,
    UCSF Stanford Health Care

Kathy Molla, R.N., M.S., Clinical Nurse Specialist,
    UC Medical Center

Jeanette Munkler, B.A., Clinical Charge Auditor,
    UCSF Stanford Health Care

Sharon Butler, R.N., Perioperative Nurse

Lucienne Maillet, D.L.S., Professor of Library and Information
    Science, Long Island University

Jean Sullivan, R.N., A.N.P., Ed.D., Associate Professor,
    San Jose State University, School of Nursing

Rhonda Jeffrey, Operations Specialist,
    UCSF Stanford Health Care

Bonnie Bialy, Senior Patient Financial Advocate,
    UCSF Stanford Health Care

TABLE OF CONTENTS

INTRODUCTION

Knowledge is Power: How to Protect Yourself

"*You need surgery.*" For many of us, hearing these simple words in our doctor's office induces a host of reactions, from feelings of helplessness to outright panic. And no wonder. Every week the newspaper headlines and TV news reports recount the latest appalling tales of medical errors and malpractice. We hear stories of bungled surgeries — healthy limbs or organs (everything from kidneys to breasts) opened and removed by mistake; serious medication errors; negligent postoperative care. According to the Harvard School of Public Health, hospital-related errors kill an estimated 180,000 Americans each year.

Of course, not every surgical procedure has such dire consequences. In fact, the vast majority of patients will have a normal, uneventful surgical experience and resume their regular lives with no problems. Still, with health care services undergoing dramatic restructuring, and cost-cutting the order of the day, today's health care consumer cannot afford — in any sense of the word — to be complacent.

In the future more and more people will be faced with the prospect of surgery. An estimated 50 million operations are performed in the United States each year; of these, approximately 80 percent are considered elective. It's shocking to note that statistically, the rising number of surgeries can be attributed not to the population growth, but rather to an increase in the number of *surgeons*. Some critics have claimed that from 10 to 25 percent of all surgeries — from hysterectomies to knee procedures — may actually be unnecessary, exposing millions of people to needless risk.

Whether you've been told you need surgery or you're contemplating an elective procedure you probably have many questions. You may also be wondering whether there's anything you can do to improve the odds that your surgical experience will be successful.

There are steps you can take as a health care consumer to protect yourself and ensure the best possible outcome. Arming yourself with knowledge — and then remaining vigilant throughout the duration of care — is the best way to protect yourself and your loved ones.

We wrote *Surgery: A Patient's Guide from Diagnosis to Recovery* to provide a compendium of consumer-oriented information on the topic of surgery — everything you need to know as a patient, from the moment you receive your diagnosis to the day to leave the hospital and continue the recovery process at home.

- *How to interview and choose a surgeon*
- *How to get a second opinion*
- *How to find out more about the surgical procedure*
- *How to prepare for surgery*
- *What actually goes on in the operating room*
- *Types and risks of anesthesia*
- *Common postoperative experiences*
- *What to expect on the nursing unit*
- *Post-discharge care*
- *Insurance and financial considerations*

We hope the information contained in this book will help answer your questions and alleviate any initial anxiety you may have about your operation. We wish you good health and a positive surgical experience.

CHAPTER ONE

You Need Surgery—Now What?

Scenario

"Your test results are back from the laboratory. The doctor would like to see you in his office this afternoon. Can you be here by 3?" You wonder, "What did the tests show? Is it serious? Will I need surgery?"

You enter the doctor's office 20 minutes early, check in, and perch on the edge of your chair. You grab a worn copy of your favorite magazine and begin leafing through the pages. Finally, the nurse comes to the waiting room door and calls your name. You toss the unread magazine onto the coffee table and follow her down the hallway into the physician's private office.

"The doctor will be right with you. Please take a seat," says the nurse as she exits the room. You scan the doctor's office. Framed diplomas and certificates cover one wall. Books and journals neatly fill several bookshelves, and his wooden desk is piled high with stacks of papers and folders.

The doctor enters and settles into his big leather chair, picks a folder from the top of the pile, and spreads it open. Your eyes dart to the folder and then to your doctor's face. He smiles reassuringly and says, " I've reviewed the results of the tests done last week, and it seems you're going to need an operation to relieve those symptoms that have been bothering you."

An operation. You take a deep breath. "I was afraid of this," you say. "So, what happens next?"

Stop. Right now, when your stress level is high, it's very easy to forget the details of a conversation. Especially when the conversation is about something as frightening as surgery on your body. Your physician has scheduled this time to spend with you. You have his undivided attention. Don't waste the opportunity to gather information and have your questions answered.

If you're reading this book prior to your appointment, come prepared with our checklist and a pencil. Or, ask for a notepad and pencil. Notes taken during this conversation with your physician will help you organize your discussion and think of additional questions. They also give you a record to review if you choose to discuss your condition with concerned family and friends.

We suggest you ask the following basic questions. If you think of others as you interview your doctor, ask them. Remember, no question is too dumb or inappropriate. This is your body you are making decisions about.

1. What has gone wrong with my body? Is it serious?
2. How does this differ from normal body functioning?
3. What causes this problem and is it common?
4. Was this problem caused by something I did? (Perhaps some heavy lifting, over-exercising, or certain foods I ate?)
5. Are there nonsurgical alternatives that might make me better?
6. What does the surgery involve?
7. What results can I expect from this surgery?
8. Will I need time off work?
9. What will my after surgery (postoperative) recovery be like?

10. Will I need pain medication or help at home?
11. What will happen if I delay making my decision to have surgery?

There are a few things to keep in mind as you discuss these questions with your doctor. Let's consider them further.

Question 1: What has gone wrong with my body?

Question 2: How does this differ from normal body functioning and is the difference serious?

These questions can be answered together. Your doctor will explain how the human body normally works, and then explain how your problem affects normal function and how seriously this affects your health. If the explanation is unclear, or if the medical words are too difficult to understand, ask your doctor to restate the sentences in plain English. Physicians speak in medical terms so frequently they often don't realize they may be using terms that are foreign to their patients.

Question 3: What causes this problem and is it common?

Question 4: Was it caused by something I did?

Again, these two questions go hand in hand. Sometimes problems are caused by the patient's lifestyle or habits. For example, it is generally accepted that smoking causes lung disease. Other times there is no connection between lifestyle and health problems. An example of a disease with no known connection to one's lifestyle is inflammation of the appendix (*appendicitis*). It's helpful for you to know if your problem was caused by something you did. If this is behavior you can control, you may improve your health by changing your habits.

Question 5:   Are there nonsurgical alternatives that might make me better?

Some problems may be addressed by either an operation (surgical intervention) or a treatment that does not require an operation (nonsurgical intervention). The nonsurgical intervention is often referred to as a conservative approach. Ask your physician to explain all of your options — both surgical and nonsurgical — for resolving your problem. As he explains each choice, ask him to outline the benefits and risks (pros and cons) of each one. Finally, ask him what he considers to be your best option and why he thinks it is the best choice for you.

An example of a problem that might be treated with either elective surgery or a nonsurgical treatment is gallstones. If the stones in your gallbladder cause you to have nausea, vomiting, and diarrhea whenever you eat fatty foods, your physician may recommend removal of your gallbladder and the accompanying stones (a procedure known as cholecystectomy).

He might also tell you that the other option is to alleviate your symptoms by carefully watching your diet and avoiding fatty foods. Watching your diet may not cure your gallstones, but it may relieve your symptoms.

Another medical condition where the patient may be offered a choice between elective surgery and a nonsurgical intervention is continuous, severe back pain. Some physicians prefer a conservative approach, which includes bed rest, use of traction, positioning devices, muscle relaxants, physical therapy, and pain medication. Other physicians will recommend an operation because they believe that while nonsurgical intervention may offer temporary relief, back problems usually reoccur. These physicians maintain that the best treatment is the more permanent cure a surgical procedure will provide.

4

Question 6: What does the surgery involve?

Your primary care physician will be able to give you basic information about your operation, but you might want to save the more detailed questions for your surgeon. In Chapter 4 we provide a comprehensive list of questions for your surgeon.

The basic questions concerning surgery you want answered by your primary care physician are the following:

- What will the surgery repair or replace?
- How soon will I need to schedule my operation?
- Which surgeon does he recommend? Why?
- Do I have the option of having my surgery in a free-standing ambulatory surgery center, or will I be admitted to the hospital?

Question 7: What results can I expect from my surgery?

It's very important to know all the expected results, outcomes, or ramifications of the recommended surgery before you make an informed decision. It's critical to understand the consequences if you decide to have any type of surgery.

An example: a very successful businesswoman was told she needed to have a bunion removed from her foot (*bunionectomy*). The adjoining joint on her toe had arthritis, and the doctor suggested removing the inflamed joint to relieve her arthritis pain. Without asking additional questions, she agreed to have the arthritic joint removed. Unfortunately, she didn't ask what the outcome of this additional surgery would be. She discovered after the operation, that the shortened toe affected her gait and impaired her ability to wear a normal dress shoe. Today she can tolerate wearing only tennis shoes. Picture her in an elegant silk party dress or impeccably tailored wool business suit wearing her ever-present tennis shoes, and you realize the permanent impact this "minor" additional surgery had on her life.

Question 8: Will I need time off from work or someone to care for the children?

You should ask how much time off you will need, both before and after your surgery. Until recently, patients were admitted to the hospital the day before their operation. This allowed them to have all the necessary blood tests, urine tests, and X-rays completed just prior to surgery. With today's emphasis on cutting the cost of health care, most patients have their preoperative laboratory tests and X-rays done in their physician's office or during prior appointments in a hospital's laboratory, X-ray departments, and admissions testing center.

Question 9: What will my recovery be like? Will I need help at home?

Early discharges are becoming increasingly common in today's managed care dominated health care market. Operations that used to require a few days' hospitalization for recovery are now considered same-day or outpatient surgeries. Ask your physician how much pain you will experience, what your pain medication requirements will be, what bandages (or dressings) your wound will need, and if you will require the services of a home care visiting nurse. Many hospitals and surgical centers now have registered nurses on staff who will make a house call and help you as you recover from your operation.

Question 10: What will happen if I delay making my decision to have surgery?

There are three categories of surgery: *emergent*, when the problem is life-threatening and the patient needs surgery immediately; *urgent*, when the problem should be dealt with within the next 12 to 24 hours; and *elective*, when the surgery can be done at your convenience and only if you choose to have the operation.

Emergent surgeries must be done quickly because the patient's problem is considered an emergency. In other words, the situation is either life-threatening and may kill the patient, or the problem will continue to rapidly worsen until it causes serious damage or cripples the patient. Some examples of emergent surgical conditions include a weakened, bulging area in a large blood vessel (*aneurysm*) that may burst and result in fatal blood loss, or a serious chest injury that interferes with breathing. If your doctor tells you your situation is emergent, he is telling you that ignoring it or delaying treatment may result in serious consequences, including permanent disability or death.

Illnesses or injuries requiring urgent surgery include such conditions or medical problems as an inflamed appendix, ectopic pregnancy (tubal pregnancy) or a broken hip that needs pins placed in order for the bone to heal correctly. In urgent cases, the surgery is necessary but the patient requires some minimal preparation and a few hours' delay will not be dangerous.

Elective surgeries are not emergencies. They do not need to be done quickly, and sometimes the problem may be remedied with nonsurgical treatments. You have a choice (or may "elect") whether or not to have the surgery. If you do decide to have the surgery, you may choose when to schedule the operation.

7

Examples of elective surgery include some types of joint replacements or cosmetic surgery like face lifts.

Remember: for most people, surgery is a major event. A person can never gather too much information or ask too many questions when making difficult choices that affect one's life and the lives of family and friends.

The questions we suggest will help you gather the basic information you and your loved ones need in order to make good decisions about your health care. Each question and the associated subjects will be discussed in much more detail in the following chapters.

CHAPTER TWO

How To Insure Your Financial Safety: Understanding Your Health Plan

Health care coverage used to be fairly simple and straightforward. An individual went to work for a company, and that company (or employer) provided health care coverage that was offered by an insurance company. The health care (or medical) coverage was part of the employee's larger benefit package that also included life insurance, a retirement plan, and vacation pay. The employer typically bore the expense for all these benefits. Health care coverage usually had two distinct expenses that employees were responsible for paying out of their own pockets: an annual *deductible* that the employee paid before the insurance company would begin paying for medical services, and *coinsurance*, a small percentage of the total bill that the employee would pay any time he or she received care from a medical provider. In short, employees and their families sought medical care with any doctor or hospital when they thought they were sick and the bills were paid by the insurance company. Most people had little reason to think about the process of receiving medical care.

Today health care coverage can feel like an enormous labyrinth as we face choices, acronyms, and rules. There are managed care plans and traditional indemnity insurance, *health maintenance organizations* (HMOs) and *primary care physicians* (PCPs), gatekeepers and open enrollment periods. New employees in a company receive brochures from all the different health plans the company offers, sometimes as many as five or six. The employee is then faced with assessing the different levels of coverage offered by each plan (does the plan cover routine office visits? Prescriptions? Immunizations? Annual gynecological visits?). The employee needs to assess the different out-of-pocket expenses for care through each of the plans (is there a copayment for the office visit or is there an annual deductible with coinsurance?); and the various rules (is there a *gatekeeper* — a primary care physician through whom an HMO participant must go for referrals to make sure medical care is paid for by the HMO? Do visits to specialty physicians require a referral?). The employee also should investigate the different monthly premium amounts with a breakdown of how much the employer will pay and how much the employee must contribute (employee only? employee and spouse? Employee and dependent child(ren)? Employee, spouse and dependent child(ren)?

Escalating Health Care Costs

The escalating cost of health care has been the major impetus for the dramatic changes we see today in health care coverage. In the United States there is a long history of steadily increasing public and private expenditures for health care services. In 1960 health care expenditures were $26.9 billion, 5.1 percent of the gross domestic product (GDP). By 1980 they had increased 820 percent to $247.3 billion, 8.9 percent of the GDP, and in 1990 rose to $699.5 billion and 12.2 percent of GDP. In 1996 health care expenditures broke the one trillion dollar mark, however, as a percentage of GDP they remained at 13.6 percent where it had been since 1993 (Health Care Financing Administration [HCFA], 1998).

This is how the monies used to flow in the health insurance system:

- Employer paid premium to insurance company to cover employee
- Employee sought medical care from any physician or is hospitalized
- Physician or hospital sent their bill to the insurance company
- Insurance company paid the physician or hospital, sometimes at a pre-negotiated discount

A similar system was used to provide health care coverage for individuals who had retired from the workforce. Medicare was introduced in the mid-1960s to provide health care coverage for persons over age 65 (and was later expanded to include long-term disabled persons). Like the system for the employed, Medicare was designed to offer health care coverage to enrollees with a reimbursement arrangement with the physicians and hospitals.

However, in both the private and government systems the costs of health care continued to increase, as did the use of medical services. Combined with this was a significant rise in the number of elderly people with Medicare coverage and, by the late 1970s, these factors led the government to face Medicare expenditures far exceeding their budgeted amounts. In an effort to control these budget overruns Congress reduced the amounts they paid hospitals for care provided to patients with Medicare, but by fiscal year 1982 the aggregate Medicare/Medicaid underpayment to hospitals had still reached nearly 6 billion dollars (Hall, 1989).

In an attempt to begin controlling these costs Medicare introduced a new hospital payment system in 1983. This system, still in effect today, is a prospective payment system that pays hospitals a flat amount (*or case rate*) based on the patient's diagnosis. *Diagnosis related group (DRG)* payments assign an expected length of stay in the hospital for each procedure, and the hospital receives a lump sum payment for that procedure. This system is designed to provide some financial incentive for the hospital to provide the most appropriate care while managing the costs. The incentives work as follows: if the patient recovers quickly and is ready to be discharged sooner than the expected length of stay, then the theory is that the hospital will benefit because it will still receive the payment that was based on a longer length of stay. The system discourages hospitals from keeping patients unnecessarily because it will not make additional payments for a length of stay beyond the assigned number of days.

DRG-based payments are one means to manage the costs of health care. Today the term *managed care* is widely used to refer to the growing types of health plans that have some financial incentives in place designed to control costs. Managed care plans use at least one and usually all three of the following features:

- Contracts with a limited number of physicians, hospitals, and other health care providers
- Compensation to its providers in such a way that incentives are provided to control health care costs
- Required use of utilization review to control unnecessary use of health care services

Although many people are newly acquainted with the idea of managed care through the health plans their employer presently offers, managed care itself is not a new concept. Henry J. Kaiser was a West Coast shipyard and steelmill owner who, in 1938, was awarded the contract to build the Grand Coulee Dam. Kaiser hired a young physician, Sidney Garfield, who provided health care services to the dam workers and their families for 50 cents a week per adult and 25 cents per child. By World War II the concept was expanded to Kaiser shipyard and steelmill workers (Bettinger, 1994). Soon Kaiser not only had its own physicians, it also had its own hospitals and in essence became the first group model HMO in the United States.

By 1998 Kaiser was the largest single managed care organization in the country, with 9.2 million members. The American Association of Health Plans (1997) reports that over 150 million Americans are enrolled in network health plans (which include HMOs, *preferred provider organizations {PPOs}*, and *point-of-service {POS}* programs). Over 80 million of those people are reported to be enrolled in HMOs alone (National Committe for Quality Assurance,1998).

What does managed care mean to the average consumer?

Most employers contribute to the monthly price (or premium) that the health plans charge to provide health care coverage. However, today it's rare to find an employer who does not require the employee to make a small, or often a large, contribution to the employee's share of the premium. This employee contribution came about for two primary reasons:

1) When health care premiums began to steadily increase, requiring the employee to share in the cost of the health plan became one way for the employer to control expenses.

2) Payment of a portion of the premium encourages employees to become active participants in the health care delivery system. This investment in the system is particularly advantageous as employees evaluate the pros and cons of managed care plans.

Managed care plans offer lower premiums than traditional insurance, and sometimes there are substantial differences in the premiums. Additionally, competition among managed care plans is fierce in many markets and one sure way to increase enrollment is to offer premiums lower than one's competitors. Unfortunately, people who choose their health plan based solely on price are often the ones who are most dissatisfied because they do not understand how to receive medical care within the new health plan. (Generally, the lower-priced plans have fewer benefits and greater restrictions. So, a consumer who makes their decision based solely on price without analyzing the services provided, restrictions, and methods of gaining authorization, etc.,may be disappointed with the new health plan.)

In addition to the low monthly premiums, managed care plans offer rich benefit packages, often including eye exams, immunization, prescription drug coverage, preventive care, and gynecological care. The cost for receiving services is then a nominal *copayment* (a flat amount), lower than the *coinsurance* (percentage of total bill) associated with receiving care in a traditional insurance plan. HMOs believe that by providing and encouraging preventive care at a reasonable cost to you they will, in the long run, be able to keep you healthier.

Consumers today usually have the choice of one or more of the following types of managed care plans when selecting their health plan coverage:

HEALTH MAINTENANCE ORGANIZATION (HMO):

An HMO is a health plan offering comprehensive health care provided by a panel of hospitals, physicians, and other health care providers. HMOs have several key components:

- Wider range of covered services, including preventive care (immunizations, well-child care, annual gynecological visits), prescriptions, and routine eye exams.

- Members must choose a primary care physician (PCP) — an internist, family practitioner, pediatrician, or general practitioner — who will provide, coordinate, or authorize all of their health care. PCPs are often referred to as gatekeepers since members must go through them to ensure that medical care is paid for by the HMO.

- PCPs are generally reimbursed on a pre-paid basis, while specialist physicians, hospitals, and other providers are reimbursed at a reduced rate of payment based on a pre-determined fee schedule.

Rather than paying coinsurance, members pay a flat nominal amount, called a copayment, when receiving care. Copayments to the PCP are often between five to $15, while copayments to the specialist are slightly higher. Emergency room copayments are usually between $25 and $50, but many plans waive them when the patient is admitted. There may also be a copayment for hospital admissions depending upon the level of coverage the employer chooses. The higher the copayments, and the more services having copayments associated with them, the lower the monthly premium.

THERE ARE THREE MODELS OF HMOs.

STAFF:

An organized prepaid health care system delivering health services through a salaried physician group employed by the HMO. Kaiser is the most famous staff model HMO.

GROUP:

An organized prepaid health care system contracting with one independent group practice to provide health services.

INDEPENDENT PRACTICE ASSOCIATION (IPA):

An organized prepaid health care system contracting directly with physicians in independent practice, and/or with one more multispecialty group practice(s) to provide health services.

PREFERRED PROVIDER ORGANIZATION (PPO): A PPO is a health plan having contracts with a large network of physicians, hospitals, and other health care providers at discounted rates. They are called preferred providers because when the member uses their services most of the bill is paid for by the managed care plan. With a PPO there is no gatekeeper and the member may elect to see any health care provider. However, those members deciding to go to a doctor who does not participate with the PPO will have to pay more money out-of-pocket.

POINT OF SERVICE ORGANIZATIONS (POS): In a POS plan members are enrolled in an HMO or PPO and receive the high level of benefits those plans offer as long as they use the proper health care providers and procedures. However, in a POS plan members also have the option of self-referring to any health care provider outside of the HMO or PPO, but will have to pay a much higher out-of-pocket amount.

HMOs are the most restrictive managed care plans, but also offer the highest level of benefits both in terms of the amount you must pay out of pocket and the covered services (preventive care, prescriptions, etc.). Point of service plans are the least restrictive and most flexible managed care plan, and PPOs fall between the two.

How do I know which plan is best for my needs?

Managed care plans offer excellent benefits at reasonable prices, but to accomplish this there are restrictions about how a patient receives care. HMOs in particular have specific procedures that must be followed in order for care to be paid for by the HMO, and it's important with any managed care plan that one understand what one is choosing before making a decision. HMOs are not for everyone, but many people do not look beyond the low monthly premiums. Unfortunately, when a medical situation arises and it's time to receive medical care, the people who don't understand their plan are the ones who will find themselves either unhappy with their plan or, in some cases, having to pay large sums of money out of pocket because they didn't follow the HMO's rules.

Many factors should be considered when evaluating the health plans available through an employer. Plans should be reviewed in detail. Married employees should discuss options with their mates in order to be able to make informed decisions or to be more satisfied with their health care coverage.

To begin the process consider the following issues:

How much will I have to pay in monthly premiums for each of the plans my employer offers?

Many employers provide a grid outlining the different health plans and their associated premiums. The premiums are based on tiers, and usually include some variety of the tiers outlined below, with premiums lowest for the employee only and highest for the employee, spouse, and child(ren).

- Employee only
- Employee and spouse

- Employee and dependent child(ren), and
- Employee, spouse and dependent child(ren)

What health care services are covered with each of the plans?

To assess the services covered by each plan first determine which health care services are important to you and your family. Consider issues such as these:

- Do I have young children?
- Am I pregnant or planning to start a family?
- Do my dependents or I have a chronic illness requiring ongoing care?
- Do my dependents or I have disabilities that require ongoing care?
- Do any of us have a pre-existing condition (a condition that began before the day coverage would begin) that might be excluded, or for which coverage might be limited?
- Am I or any of my dependents presently seeing a mental health provider?
- Do I travel frequently?
- Do I have dependents away at college or boarding school?
- Do I take any medications regularly (including birth control pills, blood pressure medication, etc.)?

Once you answer these and other questions of concern to you and your family, carefully review the benefits offered by each of the plans. Not sure if something is covered, or to what extent it's covered? Call the member services department of the plan and ask. Be sure to also ask them where in the printed materials you can review documentation verifying that the service is covered.

Which doctors, hospitals, and other health care providers participate with each of the plans?

If you're considering a plan that has a limited panel of providers it's important to look through the directory carefully and ask yourself the following questions:

Do I have an established relationship with a primary care physician (family practitioner, internist, pediatrician, general practitioner)? If so, is that physician listed in the health plan's provider directory?

If your doctor is on the list consider calling the doctor's office if you are thinking about joining the health plan and ask whether or not they are happy with the plan, and if they will continue to participate in it. Also check to see if the doctor is taking new HMO patients. Some close their practices to members from certain HMOs, and although they would probably make an exception for an existing patient, it's important to know this ahead of time.

If my primary care physician is NOT listed in the directory, am I willing to find a new one?

HMOs have a careful screening process for new physicians who join their plan. Physicians must meet certain criteria in order to be accepted. In addition to education, licensure, and certification requirements, the HMOs may also consider whether or not they have coverage when the office is closed and how many days and hours they are open during the week. HMOs can assist you in selecting a physician from their panel, and can answer questions you have about physicians you're interested in, including where they went to school, the hospitals they admit to, whether or not they're board certified, what their office hours are, etc. (*See Chapter 4 for additional information on choosing a physician*).

Am I currently receiving ongoing care from a specialist physician (cardiologist, orthopedic surgeon, ophthalmologist, obstetrician, etc.)? Is that physician in the directory? Am I willing to change physicians?

Have I had surgery or received care in the past from a specialist physician, and would I want to see that same physician again if the same or another problem occurred in the future?

If you see that your specialist physician is participating with the health plan and listed in the directory, it's important to remember that participation alone does not mean that your primary care physician will automatically refer you. If it is a condition that the primary care physician can treat, you may not be referred even if your preferred specialist participates.

Do I prefer to use a specific hospital in the event that I have to be hospitalized? Is that hospital included in the provider directory?

When choosing their managed care plan, people without existing medical conditions rarely plan to get sick. However, a person who is now healthy may at some time in the future find that they have a minor, or even serious, illness. While the threat of illness is not usually a prevailing factor in choosing a managed care plan, it is a good idea to look over the managed care plan's complete physician and hospital listing and see which hospitals and physicians participate. Ask yourself the following questions:

If I were diagnosed with cancer, does the hospital in my community that specializes in cancer treatment participate in the managed care plan?

If I were to develop a heart condition, do the well-known cardiology groups in town participate in the plan?

If I am pregnant or have small children, does the local children's hospital participate?

Certainly one cannot imagine all the conditions that might occur, but it's worth a cautious review of the hospital and physician listing to keep some of these considerations in mind. If you don't know who specializes in cancer treatment, or who the well-known cardiology groups are, ask your family physician, or call the local medical society (listed in the phone book). Or, ask friends, neighbors, or colleagues. If you know someone who works in or with the medical profession, ask them.

Determining the policies and procedures for receiving care from each plan

In order to limit costs managed care plans exercise tight control over the health care system. It's important to fully understand how each plan you're considering works, and what process you'll need to go through to receive care. The answers to the questions below can usually be found in the materials distributed by the plan, or sometimes employers will prepare a summary page comparing these procedures among each of the plans. You may also speak directly with your human resources manager to obtain answers, or call the member services department with the health plan (the phone number should appear in the plan materials).

Do I have to select a primary care physician?

In an HMO, and in most managed care plans, you must select a primary care physician (PCP) from internists, family, or general practitioners, pediatricians and, in some plans, gynecologists. The HMO has a provider directory listing all of its primary care and specialist physicians, usually broken down into geographic areas. Each family member must select a PCP who will provide for, or coordinate, all of the care to be received through the health plan. Each family member may select a different PCP. A pediatrician may be selected as a child's PCP, with an internist or family or general practitioner for the adult family members. As stated earlier, PCPs are sometimes referred to as gatekeepers because they are your first point of contact for all services within the HMO system.

Can I change my primary care physician? How do I do that? How often can I change?

Yes, you can usually always change your PCP. Contact your HMO to find out what you need to do in order to change your PCP. Some plans require that you complete a change form, and the change becomes effective the first day of the next month as long as they receive the change form by a certain deadline. One of the philosophies of an HMO is that the client develops a relationship with a PCP who knows the person and manages all aspects of care.

If you change PCPs frequently the HMO may contact you to discuss whether the plan is meeting your needs and explore why you haven't established an ongoing relationship with a PCP.

If I want to see a specialist, does my primary care physician have to refer me?

Your PCP will generally refer you to a specialist physician if you have a medical condition that is best treated by a specialist, or one this physician is not trained to care for. Just because you might want to go see a dermatologist for a skin condition, your PCP does not have to authorize that visit if it's something that dermatologist is not qualified to treat. If you have a highly restrictive plan, such as an HMO, your PCP has to give you a referral to a specialist physician in order for the HMO to pay for the visit to the specialist. If you decide to see a specialist without a referral, the visit will be considered unauthorized and the specialist can ask you to pay at the time of the visit. If you feel you should have been referred to the specialist by your PCP, you should talk with the member services department to discuss your specific situation and what recourse you have.

What services are listed under *exclusions* by the plan?

Be certain to review the exclusions carefully and make sure they don't include any services you are currently receiving or think you might need in the future. Exclusions can include: rehabilitation or rehabilitative care, services or procedures that are experimental or investigational in nature, cosmetic procedures, and *in vitro* fertilization.

How does the plan define an emergency?

Each plan may define an emergency slightly differently, but generally a medical emergency is defined as a condition requiring immediate medical attention to prevent death or disability due to a sudden trauma or illness.

If my primary care physician office is closed can I go to the emergency room or urgent care center nearest me?

Managed care plans discourage the use of emergency rooms (ER) as a place to receive non-emergent care because emergency room care is very costly. They discourage unnecessary use of the ER by imposing high copayments for emergency room care (unless you are admitted directly from the ER, in which case the copayment is usually waived) and by reviewing ER records to be sure that your condition meets their definition of an emergency. If your condition does not meet their approved criteria, you may be responsible for the entire amount of the ER bill. Be clear in your understanding of how the plan defines covered emergency room care, and understand what you should do after hours and on weekends when your PCP office is closed.

If I'm admitted to the hospital because of an emergency do I have to call the health plan and let them know? How soon do I have to call?

Does the plan require a second surgical opinion before they will pay full benefits for my surgery?

What happens if I need blood work or an X-ray? Can this be done in my primary care physician's office, or do I have to go somewhere else to have this done?

Does the plan cover immunizations, well child care, gynecological visits, or prescriptions?

Are home care and skilled nurse care covered? Is there a limit on the number of days or visits?

Is durable medical equipment (wheelchairs or crutches, for example) covered? Is there a maximum amount that will be paid?

What are the benefits for mental health? How many outpatient visits are covered per year? Do I have to have a referral from my PCP?

What do I do if I'm traveling out of the area and become ill?

If I'm unhappy with the plan when can I change plans?

Employers offer what is referred to as *open enrollment* on an annual basis. Once you make your selection of a health plan you will be committed to that plan until the next open enrollment period. Open enrollment periods are usually 12 months apart.

What is the grievance process with the plan?

All managed care plans are required to have a grievance procedure for complaint resolution. You may want to know how complaints are handled in advance of choosing a plan.

Is there a body that oversees managed care organizations? How can I obtain information about the managed care plans that I'm considering?

The National Committee for Quality Assurance (NCQA) reviews and accredits those managed care plans that meet its standards. In order to receive accreditation a managed care plan must pass a rigorous review in which the NCQA judges it on 50 different characteristics. While some plans are still waiting to be reviewed by the NCQA, those that have been reviewed can be awarded the following designations: full accreditation, partial accreditation, provisional accreditation, or they may be denied accreditation. Find out whether the plans you are considering have received full accreditation from the NCQA.

Making the final decision

Once you have answers to all the questions on the previous pages you can then determine which health plan best meets most of your needs. You probably will not find one plan that meets all of your needs and will want to look at which plan meets those most important to you. Consider making a work-sheet, listing each of the available health plans across the top and your areas of concern down the side, beginning with those that are most important to you and your family (a sample work-sheet appears at the end of the chapter).

Are you most concerned about your potential out-of-pocket expense? Perhaps you have small children, therefore affordable well-child care and immunizations may be most important. Or maybe you had bypass surgery two years ago and want to use the same cardiologist as before should anything happen in the future, yet that cardiologist doesn't participate with one of the managed care plans.

Remember that the health plan you choose now is one you will have to keep for a year. You ought to be comfortable that the plan is one you may only use for occasional prescriptions, as well as for an unexpected, life-threatening illness, should one occur.

If you enroll in a managed care plan

If you make the decision that a managed care plan is the right choice for you and your family, here are some additional situations that might come up and suggestions to help you deal with them.

I want to join an HMO, but my family practitioner doesn't belong and I really want to continue seeing him.

Call your physician and ask to speak directly with him/her or the office manager. Tell them you would like to sign up with the HMO, and see if they participate in any plans. Tell them what health plans are available through your employer and find out if they belong to one of the other health plans that is being offered to you. If they tell you they are interested in joining the plan that you're considering, understand that many HMOs have full-provider networks and are not adding any new physicians. Unless you can confirm with the HMO that your physician is in their network, proceed to sign up for the HMO as if your physician is not participating.

I've joined the HMO and my PCP referred me to a dermatologist. Now I'm getting bills from the dermatologist's office and I didn't think I was supposed to.

Call the health plan's member services department and speak with a customer service representative. If you have the proper referral from your PCP and paid your applicable copayment to the specialist you should not be receiving bills for any covered services. When you speak with the member services representative be sure to record the person's name, the date of the call, and a brief description of your conversation.

I've belonged to my HMO for over two years and I received a letter from my primary care physician yesterday telling me that she was no longer going to participate in this HMO. Can I change health plans to stay with my physician?

Unfortunately, until your employer has open enrollment again (once a year) you cannot change health plans. You should receive a letter from the health plan advising you of their process for selecting a new PCP, but if you have not received one you should call the member services department directly.

My wife was diagnosed with leukemia and found out she needed a bone marrow transplant. We have researched the best transplant programs and decided we want to go to a teaching hospital on the West Coast, but our oncologist told us that the health plan is only authorizing her to go to a regional center here in our state. We don't think this is the best place for her to receive a transplant. What can we do?

Usually people are not sick when they choose their health plan and only later, after they've been diagnosed or need treatment, do they find out that their plan may have certain limitations. *Persistence and documentation* are two of the most effective techniques in resolving a situation such as this one. An initial consideration is whether the provider directory or health plan member agreement is clear about where a patient will be referred in the event that the person requires specialized care, such as a bone marrow transplant. Research this and see if it is addressed in any of the literature you received as a member of the plan.

The patient should also have a lengthy conversation with her oncologist about the regional center the health plan uses and the teaching hospital the patient wants to go to. The patient should directly ask the oncologist's opinion about which hospital offers the best outcomes, and where the patient would be referred if the health plan were not involved. If the oncologist is clinically in agreement with the patient's desire to go to the teaching hospital the oncologist may contact the health plan to discuss referral to the teaching hospital or to explore alternatives to the regional center.

Should the patient continue to feel that she wants to go to the nonauthorized teaching hospital, then she should do as much research on her options as possible. Potential resources include the local library or health library, the Internet, the library of the nearest medical school, the teaching hospital where she wants to be treated, and medical associations involved with her specific disease. If, through her research, she compiles information demonstrating that the hospital she wants to use has better outcomes or specializes in that particular kind of transplant, then she should call the medical director of the health plan and discuss the health plan's decision. She should also ask the medical director if there is also a process for appealing this decision and be persistent in following up.

The patient should also talk with the human resources director or president of the company that provides her health care coverage. Since the employer is the purchaser of the health coverage, the employer is viewed as a client of the health plan and a company representative may be able to communicate more effectively with the health plan about its decision and also be able to explore alternatives.

Many health plans have extensive programs in place for specialized procedures such as transplantation and use only a limited number of hospitals, which are well defined in the provider directories and other health plan literature. But not all health plans have this, and if you are unclear as to how a decision was reached regarding where you are being referred, or if you have information supporting better results from another transplant program, you should talk with the health plan representative until you have a clear understanding of their decision and how it was reached. Be sure to keep concise notes including names and

dates of all the people you speak with, and copies of any correspondence. Don't hesitate to go to the top of the organization if
that's what it takes to get an answer.

Healthy, Wealthy and Wise

Managed care is a reality. Despite its critics, more than 55
percent of the population in the United States was insured by
some type of managed care plan in 1998. In addition to the
increasing number of employers who are using some type of
managed care plan, now Medicare and Medicaid are also
enrolling their members in managed care plans in an effort to
control costs.

Given these trends, it's important to figure out how you can
make managed care work for you, and how you can work with
managed care. In order to be a satisfied consumer you must be an
informed consumer when choosing a health plan for you and
your family. You need to know how much it's going to cost you
out-of-pocket, how to receive care in the managed care system,
and understand what is and what is not covered. Managed care
is all about trade-offs, and many people fail to acknowledge this.
If you go into a managed care system because of the low premiums and limited out-of-pocket expenses, yet expect the unlimited freedom of choice that comes with traditional indemnity
insurance, you are likely to be very unhappy. Conversely, if you
recognize that the lower premiums, limited out-of-pocket
expenses and rich benefit package mean that you will have to
adjust to a different health care delivery system, then you can
make the most of your managed care experience.

The keys to making managed care work for you include:

- Understanding your family's health care needs and your own
- Determining how each health plan you are considering meets your needs

To assist you in evaluating your family's needs and the health plans your employer offers, see the "Health Care Coverage Family Worksheet" and "Health Plan Overview" on the following pages. These tools can give you an idea of the types of issues to consider both in determining your own needs and evaluating the different health plans.

HEALTH CARE COVERAGE FAMILY WORKSHEET

In order to assess the various health plans offered through your employer, you should first have a thorough understanding of your family's health care habits and concerns. Having the answers to these and other questions that are important to your family prior to reviewing the different health plans will help you know what's important to you and your family.

1. What premium tier will my family and I need?
    - ❏ Employee only
    - ❏ Employee and spouse
    - ❏ Employee and dependent child(ren)
    - ❏ Employee, spouse and dependent child(ren)

2. Do I have young children who would benefit from well-child coverage? ❏ Y ❏ N

3. If I don't have children, am I pregnant or planning to start a family in the near future? ❏ Y ❏ N

4. Do any of my dependents or I have a chronic illness that requires ongoing care? Do I see special physicians for this care?
    ❏ Y ❏ N

5. Do any of my dependents have disabilities that require ongoing care? ❏ Y ❏ N
    Do I see special physicians for this care? ❏ Y ❏ N

6. Do any of my dependents or I have a pre-existing condition that might be excluded or for which coverage might be limited?
    ❏ Y ❏ N

7. Are any of my dependents presently seeing a mental health provider? ❏ Y ❏ N
    Did you respond "yes" to questions 4-7? If so, you have some special considerations when reviewing the different plans and levels of coverage.

Does the plan cover the medical care that you are presently receiving?

Are there any limitations on the coverage (e.g. mental health visits limited to 20 outpatient visits per year, plan maximums for payments on orthotics and prosthetics, etc.)?

Is the physician or other health care provider that you presently see a participating provider? If not, are you willing to find a new provider?

Be sure that you have satisfactory answers to these and other questions from any plan you consider.

8. Do I travel frequently? ❏ Y ❏ N

9. Do I have any dependents away at college or boarding school? ❏ Y ❏ N

   If you responded "yes" to question 8 or 9, be sure you understand the coverage that the plan offers in these situations. Sometimes a managed care plan will limit coverage outside of your immediate area to emergency care only.

10. How much did you and your family spend on health care coverage last year? (Include premium contributions, co-insurance, deductibles, payment for non-covered services, e.g. prescriptions, etc.) _____

    _____

    _____

11. Do you or your family members take any medication(s) regularly? ❏ Y ❏ N

    Your response to question 10 will familiarize you with how much you presently spend and allow you to compare this amount with what you can expect to pay under the different plans that are available to you. Your response to question 11 will help you determine if a plan with prescription drug coverage is important.

12. Do you have an established relationship with a primary care physician? ❏ Y ❏ N
    If so, is that physician listed in the health plan's provider directory? ❏ Y ❏ N
    If the primary care physician you are seeing is NOT in the directory, are you willing to change to a new one? ❏ Y ❏ N

    This question is crucial. If your current primary physician is not listed in the provider directory of the plan(s) that you are considering, and if you are NOT willing to change physicians, then you need to determine if there is a plan that will let you stay with your current physician.

13. Are you currently receiving ongoing care from a specialist physician (cardiologist, orthopedic surgeon, obstetrician, etc.)? ❏ Y ❏ N
    Is that physician in the provider directory? ❏ Y ❏ N
    Are you willing to change physicians? ❏ Y ❏ N

14. Have you had surgery or received care in the past from a specialist physician, and would you want to see that same physician again if same or another problem occurred in the future? ❏ Y ❏ N
    Is that physician in the provider directory? ❏ Y ❏ N
    Are you willing to see a new physician? ❏ Y ❏ N

15. Do you prefer to use a specific hospital in the event that you have to be hospitalized? ❏ Y ❏ N
    Where would you want to be hospitalized if you developed a serious medical condition?_____
    Is that hospital listed in the provider directory? ❏ Y ❏ N
    Are you willing to go to another hospital? ❏ Y ❏ N

HEALTH PLAN OVERVIEW			
	HEALTH PLAN 1 WECARE HMO	HEALTH PLAN 2 SHOTSRUS PPO	HEALTH PLAN 3 GREEN SWORD
My monthly premium			
Does my primary care physician (PCP) participate?			
How much will I pay out-of-pocket to:			
See my PCP?			
See a specialist?			
Visit the ER?			
Be admitted to a hospital?			
Do I need a referral from my PCP to see a specialist?			
Are the following covered benefits?			
Prescriptions?			
Immunizations?			
Well-child visits?			
How much will each one cost me?			

HEALTH PLAN OVERVIEW (CONTINUED)			
	HEALTH PLAN 1 WECARE HMO	HEALTH PLAN 2 SHOTSRUS PPO	HEALTH PLAN 3 GREEN SWORD
Are the following benefits covered, and are there limitations (such as only X visits per year covered)?			
Home health care?			
Durable medical ?			
Skilled nursing?			
Mental health?			
Are any medical services that I require listed as exclusions?			
Do I have any condition that the plan considers "pre-existing"?			
What is the policy for receiving care at the ER?			
What is the coverage if I'm out of the area?			
Is the managed care plan accredited by NCQA?			
Would I be happy with this plan?			

CHAPTER THREE

How to Deal with Personal Issues

Scenario

A few days ago you learned that you need surgery. Although you're trying not to become too stressed about the prospect, you keep worrying. "Will I have to spend time in the hospital? Will I need time off work? I'm in the middle of a big project, what will my boss say? The car is in the garage for some major repairs — can I afford an operation right now? Who will I ask to help care for my children and pets? Will I have a big incision and scar? Is it going to be painful? How serious is this? What if something goes wrong and I don't survive the operation?"

Anxiety and fear are normal responses to impending surgery, especially if you've never have an operation before. Sometimes the unknowns can create even more fear than the realities of the situation.

Your family and friends will try to provide reassurance, support and assistance. However, some of them may make the common mistake of assuming that a minor procedure should not be as stressful as a major operation. "It's not that big an operation. Don't fret. Everything will be fine," may be the kinds of comments offered as well-intentioned but misguided support.

It's a mistake for loved ones to downplay your concern for two reasons. First, any surgery, regardless of its type or extent, creates anxiety and fear for the patient. Second, the degree of anxiety that you and others experience is not necessarily proportional to the magnitude of the actual surgical procedure. For example, undergoing a simple biopsy to rule out cancer can create more anxiety and stress than having a major operation like a total hip replacement.

Even though the biopsy may only take 30 minutes under local anesthesia, the stress related to the findings can far outweigh the anxiety experienced by having an arthritic hip replaced. A new hip promises an improvement in your quality of life, you know what to anticipate postoperatively, and how to go about planning for your recovery. A positive biopsy often marks the beginning of an uncertain journey through additional tests, surgeries, therapies, and lifestyle changes.

It also isn't helpful if friends relate stories about their postoperative discomfort, the changes in their bodies, and their unexpected dependency during their postoperative recovery. If someone begins one of these tales, politely ask them to change the subject. Everyone's surgery is individual and you will seldom be able to predict your own surgical course based on another's experience.

Needless to say, any surgery is a major event in one's life. The total disruption of your normal routine – even if only for a day or two – can create significant stress for both you and your loved ones. We have identified some of patients' most common fears about surgery, and offer the following comments to help address your questions and concerns.

Separation from Family and Friends

It used to be a common hospital-wide policy to strictly enforce limited visiting hours. While inconvenient for family and friends, it was especially difficult for the patient. At the very moment when they were suffering the greatest amount of discomfort, fear and anxiety, they were left alone in a foreign environment devoid of all their usual support. They felt vulnerable and abandoned in this situation.

Fortunately, the rules regarding surgery and hospitalization have greatly changed over the past 10 years. For example, hospitals seldom have the strict patient visiting hours they once did. In fact, many hospitals allow family members to come and go at will and even provide a cot in the patient's room if a family member wishes to spend the night with the patient.

If you are being admitted for ambulatory surgery, a family member may stay with you for almost the entire time prior to wheeling you off to the operating room. The staff may ask for a few minutes alone with you so that you can change into a hospital gown, have your vitals signs taken and answer the preoperative questions in private. However, after that your family will be allowed to stay at your bedside while you wait for the anesthesiologist and the OR nurse to take you to surgery.

Don't hesitate to tell the nursing staff if you are very nervous before your procedure. They will inform the anesthesiologist who will give you a mild sedative to help you relax prior to going into the operating room.

Losing Control

Patients are often concerned about saying something they shouldn't — either while sedated or after general anesthesia. They fear the effects of the medications will make them reveal long-hidden family secrets or intensely personal thoughts.

We discussed this issue with hundreds of OR nurses, surgeons, and anesthesiologists whose combined experience equals thousands of hours in the operating room environment. Their responses always revealed the same answer: *patients under anes-thesia do not offer personal information*. Not one of them is aware of a patient ever saying something embarrassing prior to or after general anesthesia. Remember, if you are receiving general anes-thesia you will fall asleep within a few seconds of receiving your intravenous medications. Most patients, when asked to count backwards from 100, will seldom reach 96 before falling asleep.

Patients also express concern about losing control over bodi-ly functions and urinating or defecating during surgery. You need not worry about losing control of your bowel or bladder while you are on the operating room table any more than you do while you are sleeping in your own bed.

As the nurses prepare you on the morning of surgery, they will request that you use the bathroom shortly before getting onto your gurney. If you feel like urinating while on the stretch-er, it's probably due to nervousness. Your bladder is essentially empty if you just urinated in the bathroom. However, if you feel a real urgency to urinate after you are lying on your stretcher, tell one of your nurses and they will help you use the bathroom.

Experiencing Pain During Surgery

Another fear many patients express is that they will feel pain during their surgical procedure but be too medicated to communicate with their physician or the nurses. This is a "one chance in a zillion" situation. If you are under general anesthetic you will not feel anything, and if you have had a local or region-al anesthetic, you will be conscious, coherent, and able to talk with your surgeon about any discomfort you feel.

If your procedure is done under a local or regional anesthetic you may still feel pressure, tugging, pulling and touch, but not sharp pain. If the sensation from tugging and pressure bother you, a mild sedative may help make you more comfortable. If you experience sharp pain, more numbing medication will be injected into the surgical site and the doctor will wait until that takes effect before continuing with your operation.

Anesthesia

Surgical staff were aware for many years that general anesthesia was the riskiest part of any surgical procedure. The risks and safety issues associated with anesthesia have significantly lessened over the last decade. Please refer to Chapter 8 for an in-depth discussion of anesthesia.

You need not worry about awakening unexpectedly during your operation. In the operating room, an anesthesiologist is standing at the head of your bed monitoring not only your level of consciousness, but also your vital signs, response to anesthetic drugs, and every aspect of your well-being. Your anesthesiologist or anesthetist is highly skilled at continually evaluating your status and will make certain you always have enough medication to keep you comfortable or asleep during your procedure.

Disfigurement

You may experience some distressing *postoperative* changes in your body's appearance, depending upon the type of surgery you undergo. Visible scars are a common postoperative concern. For many people, any scar is upsetting, but this is especially true with any *radical dissection* (major surgical procedure that results in an extensive loss or restructuring of tissues).

Disfigurement following the loss of a significant body part, such as a breast or limb, also causes considerable anxiety and fear for patients. Fortunately, there are experts in the hospital or available through your surgeon's office that can help you deal with the emotional pain of disfigurement. There are also numerous support groups in the community, often staffed with volunteers who have experienced similar losses, that can help you work through some of your anxieties.

If you have lost a limb, artificial limbs have greatly improved within the last five years. Physical and occupational therapists will work with you to enable you to regain your independence and mobility.

Advances in surgical procedures have made it possible for patients with disfiguring surgeries and scars to regain near normal appearances postoperatively. For example, postop *mastectomy* (breast removal) patients can often choose to either have a breast implant or another surgical procedure that entails moving chest muscles into the amputated breast area, thus giving the appearance that the breast was never removed.

The science of *craniofacial surgery* has also made major strides in helping patients with facial disfigurements. Through the use of bone implants and tissue transplants, surgeons can repair major facial disfigurements.

Blood Loss

There is some amount of blood loss whenever surgery is performed. Patients sometimes fear they will lose so much blood that they will require a transfusion which may be contaminated with the hepatitis or human immune virus (HIV). Although transference of any virus is extremely rare, it's understandable why a patient would be concerned about this issue.

In response to this concern, blood banks and physicians now encourage patients to donate their own blood several weeks prior to having their surgery. Receiving your own blood is the safest of all options because it is not only a perfect match, but you know your own health history. The next best alternative is to solicit matching donors who you know personally and who can assure you of their health status. For example, a family member or friend who has not engaged in any high-risk behavior may be a good candidate. Someone who has been with the same sexual partner for many years, has not received any contaminated blood transfusions, or has not come in contact with contaminated needles also may be a good candidate for donating blood.

Coping Strategies

During our nursing careers we have discovered that most people handle the stress of surgery in two basic ways. Some cope by placing complete trust and responsibility for their well-being in the hands of their physician and hospital. They believe additional information only makes them more anxious and they prefer to react to situations as they are presented.

The second type actively seek information about their operation and inform themselves as much as possible. They deal with their anxiety by educating themselves and planning for possible situations or those aspects of their life that may be disrupted by the surgery and recovery period. Years ago, many people fell into the first group. Today, many more people are interested in actively participating in their own healthcare.

If you fall into the first group, skip ahead to Chapter 4. If you're in the second group and want to be informed and prepared for surgery in order to minimize your stress, then continue reading this chapter.

Getting Support

The extent of support or assistance you will need from family and friends will vary with the type of surgical procedure you are having, your personal level of anxiety, and your family situation. Keep in mind that like your level of anxiety, the support you need is not necessarily proportional to the extent or seriousness of your operation.

Fracturing your right arm and undergoing an operation to insert a metal plate with subsequent casting is not a serious procedure. However, it can result in you being very dependent on others for several weeks. A breast biopsy for cancer can require tremendous preoperative emotional support, but if the results are negative, you probably won't need any follow-up care or additional support.

Understanding the nature of your operation and the extent of your recovery will help guide you in beginning to plan for the level of care and support you will need postoperatively.

Issues you may have to deal with include:

- Child care
- Meal preparation
- Care of your home
- Pet care
- Home health care after discharge
- Bill payment
- Job related issues: employee benefits/rights, medical leave, orienting your temporary substitute, working from home

Sources of Support

Make a list of those you consider to be your sources of personal support. This may include family members, co-workers, friends, and members of your church.

Try not to limit your list to the one or two people that are closest to you. Depending upon your situation, you may need a great deal of support and those who are always available to love and care for you may not be able to provide the total amount of assistance you will need. They may need help to care for you.

Consider if you had a co-worker or acquaintance in crisis, would you be willing to lend a hand if asked to do so? There are many ways to help besides giving direct personal care. For example, would you be willing to cook a casserole for a family or run an errand or pick up groceries for them while doing your own marketing? If you are willing to do that for others, you can understand why others probably will not hesitate to do the same for you. Write down their name and telephone number so you can call them if you need their assistance.

Many communities have organized support groups for people with medical conditions similar to yours. Some of these organizations may be local and others may be nationally based. Your physician – or the social service department of the hospital if you are having your surgery in a hospital – can provide you with information and contacts with the community organizations. Many Internet sites are targeted to specific diseases and health conditions. Use a Web browser or search engine and type in a few key words such as your diagnosis. You can also inquire about information from the following two national organizations:

The National Health Information Center
P.O. Box 1133
Washington, DC 20013-113
800-336-4797

National Self-Help Clearing House
City University of New York
Graduate Center
33 W. 42nd Street
New York, NY 10036
212-354-8525

Family Issues

Home

Routine cleaning, laundry, watering of plants, and cooking meals may not be a problem for you postoperatively. This will be dependent upon the extent of your surgical procedure. If you think you may have difficulties, plan ahead and arrange for a housekeeping service, delivered meals, or accept a friend's offer to help. To minimize the workload on any one person, ask each friend to do one or two small chores when they stop by to visit you. Most people will be happy to wash some dishes, feed the cat, or do a load of laundry.

It's important to plan ahead for any limitations and restrictions your surgery may temporarily place on you. If you know you will not be able to navigate stairs for several weeks after your operation, and your bedroom and bathroom are on the second floor, organize a room or area downstairs to serve as your sleeping area and set up your bath in the downstairs powder room or laundry. Bring any necessary articles of clothing and personal hygiene supplies downstairs. Plan as though you will be spending several days downstairs, not just an overnight. Whatever you can remember to get downstairs before surgery is one less thing you will have to do without or depend on someone else to retrieve for you after surgery. A bed in your living room may not be the way you prefer to decorate, and your downstairs powder room may be cramped, but the convenience will far outweigh the esthetics.

Child Care

Children can be your greatest concern if you are the primary care giver in your family. If you will be severely limited postoperatively, and you have small children, it may be wise to consider hiring temporary in-home help, having the children stay several days with family or friends, or enrolling them in full days at a daycare center or camp. If your spouse or significant other comes home in the evening and is willing to take responsibility for the children, it may be best to have the children brought home after dinner time so they can see you and be reassured that you are recovering. Arranging for the children to be home for only a few hours while another adult is present may also be the best option if the patient is not the primary care giver, but needs several hours of quiet, uninterrupted rest during the day.

Turn the experience into an adventure for them. Sit with each child prior to going for your surgery and have them choose a favorite toy or two, their "security blanket," and a couple of their favorite outfits to be placed in a backpack for their adventure days which will begin the day you leave for surgery. Develop a chart to record their daily activities when they return each evening to tell you how their day went. Let them color in or "X" out the boxes as they tell you about the favorite game they played, new friends they met, new things they saw, new foods they tasted, and other highlights of their busy day. If you feel well enough to read their favorite stories to them, this is an opportune time to do so.

Pet Care

In most communities there are a variety of pet care services available. They range from kennel placement to hiring someone who will come to your home to feed, water, and exercise your pet(s). Which service you arrange to use will depend upon your ability to carry out your particular pet care routine postoperatively. Sprinkling a few flakes of food into a fish tank is considerably different than walking a frisky young puppy who weighs more than you do, or trying to open a can of cat food with one arm in a cast.

It's best to err on the side of caution and assume that any pets who require a significant amount of daily care will be more than you can comfortably handle immediately after surgery. If you live alone, and plan to continue caring for your pets yourself, anticipate the unexpected and leave a key with someone who is willing to care for your pets in the event you encounter complications that require you to spend unexpected time in the hospital. You do not want to be lying awake in the hospital worrying about your beloved pet(s).

Home Health Care

In today's managed care environment, an increasing number of surgical procedures are done on a "same day" basis, which means that patients have their surgery and go home on the same day. Even if the surgical procedure requires hospitalization, the number of days patients stay in the hospital (length of hospital stay) is decreasing. This often means patients are being discharged home with bandages, tubes, or other medical devices requiring ongoing nursing care. Many surgical facilities employ registered nurses who make house calls or home visits for their surgical patients. Hospitals often offer a similar service, either through their own home care department or in partnership with a private home care agency. Your surgeon's office staff or the hospital discharge planners can help you obtain referrals for this home care service. *(See Chapter 13, "Discharge: Going Home and Home Care.")*

Work Considerations

Once you understand your medical condition and the implications of surgery, it's time to schedule a meeting with your employee human resources (HR) department representative to discuss your medical and time off benefits.

With luck, you will have paid sick time available and, depending upon which state you live in, you may have accrued state disability income as well. If necessary, discuss whether or not your company offers family leave or a medical leave of absence. What are the requirements and procedures for requesting time off for illness or surgery? How long can you be off the job and still have your existing job held for you? What happens if you need additional time off?

During this same visit, ask to talk with someone who can advise you about your medical insurance benefits. What health care services are covered? How do you file a claim? Are there restrictions or special procedures you must follow? Does your insurance plan cover assistance at home if your surgery requires it?

When to begin and end your medical leave is dependent upon how quickly you must have your operation (is it emergent, urgent, or elective?) and the expected recovery time. If you are having an elective procedure you may want to take into consideration the status of your work environment. That is, can you wait until summer vacations are over, the busy season has ended, or your most likely substitute has been oriented to cover your duties and responsibilities? Do you want to make arrangements to work from home? How will information be transferred back and forth between your office and home? Can you arrange for e-mail access or a courier service?

You will have discussed with your surgeon whether or not you will have temporary or permanent restrictions placed upon the type of work you do. For example, a longshoreman who does a lot of heavy lifting and is going into surgery for his third inguinal hernia repair may have a permanent restriction placed on the amount of weight he may lift. On the other hand, a nurse who has a broken arm and is casted while the bone mends may be temporarily restricted to a desk job such as watching the bank of cardiac monitors in the coronary care unit. Discuss your own possible restrictions with your manager and work together to find the best solution. Keep in mind that your health and well-being are the most important issues.

CHAPTER FOUR

How to Interview and Select Your Surgeon

Scenario

Your primary care physician has recommended a surgeon to perform your operation. You are unfamiliar with this surgeon, and would like to obtain some background information about her professional history before agreeing to have her do your surgery.

Are there specific questions you should ask and have answered before making a decision? Absolutely. We recommend you prepare to interview the surgeon just as thoroughly as you prepared to interview your primary care physician. There are two very important subjects to discuss with the surgeon. The first is her credentials and experience. The second is exactly what your operation will include, the pros and cons of the procedure, and the expected outcome.

Background Information

Before beginning to research your physician's professional history, it's helpful to have a basic understanding of the traditional path of medical education in this country. Higher education begins with four years of undergraduate schooling during which students earn a Bachelor's degree. This degree frequently is in one of the sciences (biology, chemistry, etc.), but that's not always the case.

Upon completion of the Bachelor's degree, an additional four years of medical school are completed. The two major degree tracks for medical training are either medical doctor (M.D.) or doctor of *osteopathy* (D.O.). These curriculums combine classroom theory with clinical application and direct patient care. Following graduation from medical school, a year of internship is completed in a hospital. This year may be done with a surgical or a medical focus, but it is predominantly general patient care. After an internship, the physician may choose to begin a residency in a specialty area. The length of residency depends upon the type of residency (specialty area). For instance, a *pediatric* residency may require two years to complete while a *neurosurgical* residency may take seven years. A residency program affiliated with a major university and/or teaching hospital may provide a greater mix of cases resulting in a broader base of experience and academic challenge.

Physicians who wish to obtain even more education and training in a specific field, may complete a fellowship. Again, the length of the fellowship is determined by the specialty area.

All physicians also have the option of becoming board certified in their specialty area(s). This entails taking several years of additional, post-medical school education and training in their specialty area, then passing a very rigorous written and oral examination administered by a team of specialists in the field. A physician who has completed all of the required additional training, but has not yet taken the examinations is considered to be "board eligible."

It is important to note that board certification is not always necessary, nor is it an absolute guarantee of excellence. Some highly skilled physicians, with great expertise, may not have taken their board examinations. And remember, not every physician's practice requires the specialized education and training of board certification. An experienced but not board certified physician may be able to care for you quite competently, especially if your problem is not complicated or unusual. However, if you have a serious medical condition, or are not improving with the usual therapies, you might want to consider seeking out a board certified physician.

Most board certified physicians also become members of their medical specialty's societies, colleges, and academies. Physicians who meet all of that society's professional requirements are called fellows of the society and may use that designation after their names. For example, surgeons who are members of the American College of Surgeons are considered Fellows of the American College of Surgeons and will use the initials FACS after the M.D. designation. (Jane Doe, M.D., FACS). Each specialty has similar societies.

In areas with teaching hospitals, many community physicians serve as associate faculty members and full-time faculty members maintain a practice within the hospital's clinic system. Physicians who spend a portion of their time teaching are most often up-to-date with the latest technology and research in their specialty area.

Researching Your Physician

The easiest way to begin researching your physician's professional history is by using the telephone. Be prepared to tell the person answering your inquiry the following: physician's full name, address, city, and state where practicing.

- American Board of Medical Specialties: 800-776-CERT(2378). They can tell you if a physician is board certified in any specialty.

- American Board of Surgery: 215-568-4000. They can tell you if the physician is board certified.
- American Board of Anesthesiology: 919-881-2570. They can tell you if the anesthesiologist is board certified in anesthesiology.
- American Society of Anesthesiologists: 847-825-5586 They can tell you if the physician is in good standing with the college.

State Medical Licensing Board

Look in the telephone book white pages under "Government/State" for "Medical Board of Your State." In some states, they will tell you if the physician is licensed by them and carrying malpractice insurance. These are two very important pieces of information for you to obtain. A reputable physician should be licensed by the state medical licensing board and should carry malpractice insurance. Although physicians do not need malpractice insurance to provide care within their own office or office-based surgical suite, if they care for patients in a hospital they are required to carry malpractice insurance. With lawsuits so commonplace today, there are only two reasons a physician would not carry malpractice insurance: if he has had so many malpractice suits filed against him that the insurance companies refuse to sell him insurance, or if his history of malpractice suits has made purchasing insurance prohibitively expensive. In either case, lack of malpractice insurance can be a "red flag." The state medical licensing board may also tell you about any past malpractice issues, but will not give you information about pending cases.

Local Medical Society

Look in the telephone white pages under "Medical Society of Your County or City." They will tell you if the physician has joined the local medical society. Ask for the types and titles of the programs sponsored by the society to get an idea of the organization's activities and where they concentrate their resources. Ask if the physicians you are inquiring about is an active, participating member of the society.

Directories and Lists

Another place to begin researching a physician's professional history is in your local public library or health library. The reference librarians are extremely knowledgeable and can advise you about which books are available and how to use them. Most of these books are strictly for use in the library, and are not to be checked out. Come prepared with pen and paper to take notes or coins for the photocopier. If your branch does not carry these resources, ask to have them loaned from a larger branch. They are available by special order from bookstores, but some tend to be quite expensive.

1. *Board Certification Directory* This book contains information about individual physicians, indexed by general specialty or the area of the country in which he or she practices. Specific information available in this reference includes: physician name, specialty, where the medical degree was earned, type, site of internship, type, site and length of residency, type ands site and length of fellowship. It also includes the length of time the physician has been in practice and any board certifications. As is true with board certification, you will have to decide how impor-

tant the physician's number of years in practice is for you and your situation.

Generally, the younger physicians are schooled with the latest knowledge about techniques and therapies, but have limited experience. The longer established physicians are very experienced, but their familiarity with new information is dependent upon how aggressively they pursue additional educational opportunities.

In addition to the number of years in practice, another important question to ask is how many years the physician has practiced at each location. Physicians who are repeatedly accused of neglect or incompetence resulting in patient injury or death typically move from state to state in order to avoid licensing restrictions or other penalties.

States and hospitals tend to keep investigations of problem physicians with questionable behaviors very confidential. The existence of investigations, and their findings, are virtually inaccessible to medical consumers. Even if the physician has a long history of malpractice incidences or other professional problems, it can be very difficult to obtain any information.

The state is the only entity with the authority to revoke a physician's license, and it is a privilege seldom exercised. States are traditionally very reluctant to revoke a physician's license, preferring instead to require additional training or application of some other penalty or restriction. Rather than work under the restriction, the problem physician moves to another state, obtains licensure, and begins anew.

Physicians and hospitals are also very hesitant to police physician practices. Unfortunately, there are too many documented examples of dangerous physicians being found guilty of gross misconduct who are allowed to keep their licenses. Usually some kind of deal or arrangement is made to protect the physician and limit the exposure for the hospital. For example, a hospital may agree to remove from their records all references to a physician's suspension for misconduct (or activities serious enough to be considered malpractice) in return for the physician agreeing never to practice in that hospital again. Frequent, unexplained moves from hospital to hospital or state to state may be another "red flag."

2. *The American Medical Directory* contains references similar to the Board Certification Directory.

3. *The Directory of Medical Specialists* contains references similar to the Board Certification Directory.

4. *13,012 Questionable Doctors*, a directory published by the Public Citizen's Health Research Group (Washington, DC) is a state-by-state directory listing of practicing physicians who have documented incidents of incompetence or other very serious problems.

5. *The National Practitioner Data Bank*, a database established by Congress, includes pertinent professional information about physicians including education, certification, malpractice suits, and disciplinary actions. Currently this database is only available to hospitals and medical boards. Legislation has been drafted to also allow consumers to access the information.

6. *Internet databases*. Search online files from your Internet service provider for additional information and publications. Refer to your membership guide for instructions on how to search the health databases and the usage charges for each. Keep in mind that if you find a Web page for your physician, he or she probably provided the information on the Web page and it was developed as a marketing tool.

Another helpful source of information may be a nurse or physician you have a personal relationship with who is willing to either share their opinion with you or ask other health care professionals on your behalf. We find a good leading question to be "If you or your significant other needed my type of surgery, who would you refer them to?" You will want to know how the surgeon performs at a given hospital, how frequently he or she does your type of surgery, how well respected the surgeon is by physician colleagues, and the operating room nursing staff, the surgical units and the emergency department. You want to know about any questionable practice issues or problems the surgeon has had with patients. Remember, this is *very* subjective information.

You may also find it beneficial to ask friends or family members who may have been a patient of the surgeon for their opinions. It's important that this family consumer also be a savvy health care consumer By this we mean someone who made extensive inquiries and checked the physician's credentials before they allowed him to do their own operation. Just because a physician is nice does not mean the person is competent.

Once you have been able to evaluate your physician's credentials and are comfortable that this professional is among the best qualified to do your operation, you are ready to ask specific questions about the operation itself.

Additional Considerations and Questions

This preliminary meeting is also the time to ask your surgeon questions about who else will be involved in your procedure and who else may be present in the operating room during your surgery.

A routine staff of professionals is required for every surgical procedure. In addition to your surgeon, there will be a circulating nurse who manages your nursing care, and a scrub person/nurse who assists during the operation by handing the sterile instruments and equipment to your surgeon.

Several other individuals may be involved as well. Ask if there will be other doctors or surgeons assisting your surgeon. Often your surgeon will require an assistant to help with the actual surgery. This assistant can be another surgeon with the same knowledge and skills, or a nurse with specialized training to assist with your specific type of procedure. This nurse is called an RN First Assist. Also ask if there be "house staff," also known as medical students, interns, and residents. What will their roles be? Will they be allowed to do any of the procedure?

House staff are usually available to hospitals that have a relationship with a medical school and have established formal teaching programs. These individuals have already received their medical degree and are now studying in their area of specialty. They are supervised by surgeons within their specialty and cannot perform surgery independently.

Other professionals may be present in your operating room depending upon the type of surgery you're having. For example, certain surgical procedures require the use of lasers or X-rays. If you will need this special equipment, specialized technicians will be present to operate the equipment. If a certain laboratory test or pathology specimen is required, the laboratory technician or pathologist will be present to handle specimens.

Other students affiliated with medical or nursing schools are allowed in the operating room to observe. These students have very specific objectives for their observation period and are never allowed to perform unsupervised patient care.

While this is controversial, sometimes representatives from medical supply companies are allowed in the operating room. While it may seen inappropriate to have a supply company representative in the operating room , it is sometimes necessary. An example of appropriate attendance by a medical supply company representative is in the case when a new heart pacemaker is inserted into a patient. The company representative is specially trained to determine and adjust the electrical setting of the pacemaker. The representative may also be standing by with several different sizes of pacemakers, waiting until the incision is made and it can be determined what size pacemaker will be best for the patient.

Another subject to discuss with your surgeon is the type of equipment to be used during your procedure. You will also want to ask how familiar both your surgeon and the operating room staff are with use of this equipment.

There are several different pieces of equipment routinely used during every operation:

- An operating table
- Surgical lights
- Electrocautery machine
- Anesthesia machine
- Physiological monitoring devices

All operating room physicians and staff are very comfortable using these routine pieces of equipment.

The advancement of medical technology continually introduces new equipment into the operating room environment. These technologically advanced pieces of equipment can improve the surgical procedure and patient outcomes tremendously. However, with each new piece of equipment the staff must learn something new. Ask what the hospital policy is in bringing new equipment into the operating room. More specifically, ask your surgeon if she plans to use any new equipment during your surgery. If she does, ask how often she and the nursing staff have used this equipment. Ask if they have studied the equipment or had specialized training regarding the equipment.

Once you have a good understanding about the equipment to be used during your procedure, discuss any concerns you may have about its use. You are completely within your rights to challenge the use of a piece of new equipment if you are uncomfortable with it being used on you. The more information you have about your procedure and the staff the better decisions you can make about your health. Your physician should understand and support this concept.

This is also your opportunity to find out exactly what the operation includes. You will want to know:

Where will the incision be made? Ask the surgeon to draw it on your body with washable marker or to sketch it on paper.

How large will the incision be?

What will be done in the operative site (is the surgeon adding, removing, repairing, or evaluating something)?

What types of incision closure should I expect (stitches, sutures, staples, and tape are possibilities)?

Will there be bandages or drains postoperatively?

Will I need blood replacement (a blood transfusion)?

Will I require a tube in my windpipe or any other supportive technology (external heart pacemaker, intravenous "I.V." lines, etc.)?

What does the surgeon plan to do if she discovers something during my surgery? (*For example, suppose you are having a biopsy of a breast tumor. The surgeon will cut out a small section of the tumor and send it to the laboratory for a quick diagnosis while you remain asleep on the operating table. Do you want her to proceed with a breast removal (mastectomy) if the tumor is cancerous? Is it safe to wait and schedule another operation? Do you want to undergo a second operation, or would you prefer to get everything done at once? Find out what your options are and don't forget to ask about the consequences of each option.*)

Is there more than one surgical approach?

Today, many operations are performed without the traditional large incision. These operations, called endoscopic or laparoscopic procedures, are done by looking inside the body through tiny, metal scopes, the size of large drinking straws. This usually entails making three to five small incisions or puncture wounds around the surgical site. The scopes and any necessary instruments are passed through these puncture wounds and allow the surgeon to work inside the body.

This scope approach is becoming increasingly favored by patients because it results in far less discomfort, a shorter length of stay in the hospital, a faster recovery time with rapid return to normal activities, and leaves minimal scarring.

Ask your surgeon if your procedure can be done with this relatively new surgical approach. If it seems possible, ask how many of these procedures have been done by this surgeon, how patients have done postoperatively, or if they had any complications from the procedure. Some surgeons do not perform enough of these operations to maintain the high level of skill necessary for ongoing proficiency. If your surgeon has only done a dozen or so operations using the scope technique, and you wish to have your surgery done using this approach, you should consider finding another surgeon.

You can tactfully accomplish this by asking your surgeon to recommend a surgeon who is highly skilled in endoscopic work. Then tell your surgeon that since you already have established a trusting relationship, you would like your surgeon to assist with the operation. Be aware some insurance companies may refuse to pay for an assistant surgeon, which may take this option away from you if you have financial constraints and can't pay for the second surgeon with your own money.

Would a second surgeon's opinion be helpful?

Is it really necessary to get a "second opinion"? This, in most instances, is something you need to decide for yourself. If your problem is common and your symptoms straightforward, a second opinion may not be necessary. For example, if you know you have an abdominal hernia (and in many cases you can see the hernia bulge) you know that depending upon the type of hernia, your choices are to leave it alone, wear a hernia binder, or have the hernia surgically repaired. Getting a second surgeon's opinion about something so straightforward may be unnecessary.

On the other hand, if your problem is serious and the potential surgery complicated, then a second opinion can be extremely helpful. We must caution you, surgeons will occasionally disagree about diagnosis and treatment options. Always keep in mind that the final decision is yours, and the better informed you are, the better decision you will be able to make.

If you decide to seek another opinion, carefully review your insurance policy. Your policy may not pay physicians for second opinions. Or you may discover that your company actually requires a second opinion but requires that specific physicians be seen for the second opinion. It's best to speak to your insurance representative before scheduling an appointment if you have questions about how they manage second opinions.

If the cost of an additional evaluation is not an issue, seek out resources that can help you find another well-qualified surgeon to provide you with one. Ask members of your family and friends if they know of anyone who has undergone the same operation you require. Call that person and ask who performed their surgery and if they were pleased with the surgeon and the results of their operation.

Other potential resources include the referral center or health library of the local hospital. You can also call the local medical association and associations for patients with your type of problem (for example, the American Heart Association or the American Lung Association). All of these associations are usually listed in the yellow pages of the telephone book under "Associations."

Ask this second surgeon if costs can be kept down by reviewing test results and X-rays already done by your first physician. If the answer is "yes" – and it probably will be – ask that the initial test results from the physician who originally ordered them be sent to your second surgeon. This usually requires that you sign a release form and there may be several days or weeks delay in forwarding the materials. If time is short, or you are concerned about the reliability of the transfer, ask if you may hand carry your records and X-rays. In some instances you will be allowed to hand carry them to your second opinion appointment.

Do I have a choice of dates and times for my surgery?

This is an excellent time to ask your physician which days of the week he does surgery. Most surgeons are affiliated with an operating room that provides them with specific, dedicated surgical time during each week. The surgeon tries to schedule all of his patients for surgery during these reserved time frames.

If you have a particular preference for the day of your operation, bring it to your physician's attention. Many people prefer to have minor-to-moderate operations done towards the end of the week (Thursday or Friday) so they can recover over the weekend and minimize time off from work.

You may also want to discuss the time of day to schedule your operation. If you are very apprehensive, you should consider asking to have your operation begin early in the morning. Most operating rooms start their first operations at 7:15 a.m., which means the first patients have to be at the surgical center, admitting department, or operating room by 6:00 a.m. so that all the preparations can take place.

Most of the second round of operations usually begin between 9:00 a.m. and 10:00 a.m., so those patients' preparations begin at 7:30 a.m. The great advantage to being an early case is that you don't have time to get nervous. You will be busy from the moment you arrive at the hospital until you are taken to the operating room.

Ask to be referred to the hospital's patient relation's office or social service office if you live far from the hospital and discover you will need tests completed just before your operation or if you have an early start time. Some hospitals arrange discounted room rates with local hotels for their out-of-town and preoperative patients.

The following questions have already been answered by your primary care physicians. However, it is a good idea to make certain your surgeon agrees with the information you have been given. If you find any discrepancies between what your primary care physician told you and what your surgeon tells you, ask each physician to clarify the matter.

Will I need anesthesia? What type? Who will be my anesthesiologist?

See Chapter 8 for our detailed discussion of anesthesia. Ask your surgeon what type of anesthesia is preferable for you to have for the operation and why this particular anesthesiologist is being recommended. Check the anesthesiologist's credentials and ask how can you speak to the anesthesiologist if you have questions. Because they usually don't practice with set office hours, anesthesiologists can be difficult to reach.

What can I expect the results of my surgery to be?

It's very important to know all the expected results, outcomes, or ramifications of the recommended surgery before you can make an informed decision. It's critical for you to ask what the consequences will be if you decide to have any type of surgery.

Will I need time off from work or someone to care for the children?

You should ask how much time off you will need, both before and after your surgery. Until recently, patients were admitted to the hospital the day before their operation. This allowed them to have all the necessary blood tests, urine tests, and X-rays completed just prior to surgery. With today's emphasis on cutting the cost of health care, most patients have their preoperative laboratory tests and X-rays done in their physician's office or during prior appointments in the hospital's laboratory, X-ray departments, and admissions testing center.

What will my recovery be like? Will I need help at home?

Early discharges are increasingly common in the contemporary managed care or HMO (healthcare maintenance organization) dominated healthcare market. Operations that used to require a few days' hospitalization for recovery are now considered same-day or outpatient surgeries. Ask your physician how much pain you will experience, what to expect your pain medication requirements will be, what bandages (or dressings) your wound will need, if you will be requiring the services of a home care visiting nurse. Many hospitals and surgical centers now have registered nurses on staff who will make a house call and help you as you recover from your operation.

Remember, for most people, surgery is a major event. You can never gather too much information or ask too many questions when you are making difficult choices that affect your life and the lives of your family and friends.

The questions we suggest you ask will help you gather the basic information you and your loved ones need in order to make good decisions about your health care.

CHAPTER FIVE

How to Choose a Surgical Facility: Free-Standing Ambulatory Surgical Center or Hospital?

Scenario

Your surgeon has completed your preoperative examination and invited you into his office for further discussion of your upcoming operation. He reaches across his desk and hands you three brochures describing nearby facilities: the free-standing ambulatory surgery center, the community hospital, and the university medical center.

He smiles and says, "I have surgical privileges at all these facilities. Since you will be having a relatively minor procedure, I recommend using the surgery center. However, where you have your surgery is your choice. Just call my receptionist with your decision."

You thank your surgeon for the brochures, tell him you will read the literature, and promise to call his office within a few days.

How are you going to make this important decision? What facts do you need in order to make the best choice? Here's some information we think will be helpful.

SMG Marketing Group of Chicago tracks surgical trends. They predict that by the start of the next century, hospitals will have a 59 percent market share for outpatient surgeries, compared to 20 percent for free-standing centers and 21 percent for physicians' offices. Contrast that with the 72 percent of market share that hospitals held in 1992. Why is the trend towards more same day (outpatient) procedures? What makes these facilities different from each other?

Free-Standing Ambulatory Surgery Center

Free-standing ambulatory surgery center. What does that mean? You probably already know that it's a place or center for surgery, but what about the rest of the description? What is the significance of "free-standing" and "ambulatory"?

Free-standing centers are usually not physically connected to another larger facility, such as a hospital or clinic. Often they occupy a small, separate building – or the floor of an office high-rise – much like your physician's office building. They may share administration with a larger facility or they may be independent businesses. In some instances these business are run by physicians.

The word "ambulatory" refers to the type of patients who can appropriately use these centers. To have an operation done in one of these centers, one must be in good health, physiologically stable, able to move about, and require the types of surgery that do not need an overnight stay. The federal Health Care Financing Administration (HCFA), which oversees Medicaid and Medicare funding, considers surgical procedures safe for outpatient settings if they are less than 90 minutes in duration; have a recovery time of less than 4 hours; a limited blood loss and limited body cavity invasion.

If you take all this into consideration, you can visualize what constitutes a free-standing ambulatory surgery center: an independent building where short operations requiring limited recovery time, minimal blood loss, and limited body cavity penetration, are performed on patients who are otherwise healthy and are able to enter and leave the building with minimal assistance.

The free-standing ambulatory care center can offer several advantages. The controlled patient volume and independent location often mean you'll find adequate and convenient parking. The admission clerk, laboratory, operating rooms, and recovery rooms are all centrally located. There is little chance you will have to walk long corridors or navigate from the first floor to the fifth and back again. You will be able to sign in, undress, and prepare for your operation, have your procedure, recover, and meet your family all in the same centralized area.

The free-standing ambulatory surgery centers generally consist of four or five operating rooms staffed by a small and well-trained group of nurses and technicians. They're accustomed to working with the types of predictable operations or procedures the center accepts. Since their patients are healthy and the operations are not complicated, they are seldom rushed or interrupted by an emergency. You will probably find them attentive and the atmosphere warm and friendly.

Free-standing ambulatory surgery centers are able to control their costs, which may result in savings for you. For example, they don't need to maintain multiple ancillary services such as an X-ray department, social services, special laboratories, a personnel department, or even a cafeteria. Another cost saving factor is that the center is not governed or accredited by the same organization as the hospital. The accreditation process, in and of itself, is a very costly process because it requires a number of fixed expenses. Last year one large 400-bed hospital paid over $50,000 to have a survey team review the facility and its practices for accreditation. This is not an unusual fee for a large hospital to pay.

The smaller free-standing center has less overhead than a large hospital. Their procedures are done only during the day, so the higher paying evening/night shifts are not part of their expenses. They are knowledgeable about the normal timeframes and necessary supplies for the procedures they do, and can often predict your length of stay and the price of your operation. Physicians know they need to keep costs down and are much more cooperative about minimizing waste. This predictable price allows you to budget for your operation and, in many cases, make a pre-payment or total payment upon admission.

If you opt to have your procedure in a free-standing ambulatory surgery center, you will want to clarify with your physician how prepared the staff is for emergencies, and what is the procedure for transferring you to a hospital, should there be unexpected complications during your operation.

You must also be certain you have arranged for someone to drive you home after you have awakened and are discharged from the center. You will not be released to go home until you are alert and oriented with stable vital signs and no dizziness or nausea. The staff will also be certain you are able to urinate (some anesthetics may temporarily inhibit your ability to urinate) and that your pain is controlled. However, the anesthesia you received makes it unsafe for you to drive for 24 hours after your surgery, no matter how good you may feel.

Hospital-based Ambulatory Surgery Center

Hospital-based ambulatory surgery centers frequently have patient admitting criteria similar to the free-standing centers: the patient must be stable and scheduled for a procedure that does not require overnight hospital admission. The major difference is that hospital-based surgery centers are usually physically located within the hospital buildings.

Although they offer the same services as free-standing centers, these hospital-based surgery centers may not be quite as convenient as the free-standing centers. Often the hospital has renovated an existing area for the ambulatory or same-day surgery center. This means you may have to compete with all patients, employees, and visitors for space in the hospital parking area. If a dedicated entrance is not available, you must enter the main hospital with all other foot traffic.

Another inconvenience is that not all hospital-based surgery centers have dedicated admission, laboratory, and X-ray services. You may be required to register in the hospital's main admitting department, make your way to the hospital laboratory for testing, the radiology department for your X-rays, and then finally go to the surgery center for your preoperative preparation. If the signs in the hospital aren't easy to follow (and effective hospital sig-nage is often a chronic problem) you may have difficulty locat-ing these various areas. In order to allow for all the time it will take you to move between the departments, you may need to be at the hospital two or three hours prior to your scheduled operation.

You should also be aware that if the hospital has not desig-nated specific operating rooms for only ambulatory (outpatient) cases, but rather mixes both inpatient and outpatient cases into the operating room schedule, there is always the chance that an emergency will supersede or "bump" an ambulatory case. This results in unpredictable operating room times that may disrupt your plans and add to your costs.

The big advantage of using a hospital-based surgical center is the accessibility of physicians, staff, and equipment if you experi-ence some sort of emergency during surgery. If you unexpectedly have an allergic reaction to a drug, suffer cardiac arrest, or another emergency situation, there is always staff available to respond to the emergency. Once you have been stabilized, spe-cial intensive care units are nearby.

You should be aware that this 24-hour availability of emergency services contributes to the hospital's operating costs. As a result, these indirect costs far exceed the cost of operating a free-standing surgery center only eight or 10 hours per day.

In addition, surgeons working within a hospital system tend to be less conscientious about controlling their use of supplies and equipment. They are accustomed to having unlimited quantities of the items they need to do their surgeries. You should compare the prices of your hospital-based surgery center to the free-standing center costs. Sometimes the hospital has established a pricing structure that makes it competitive with the free-standing center but other times it may charge more to help cover these additional expenses.

When you are given a price quote from a surgical facility, document the date, time, and name of the person who gave you the information. Make certain you know exactly what is covered by the quoted price and what is not covered (and those additional charges) so you can make accurate comparisons. Remember, in most cases the price quoted is only for the facility fee. It usually does not include the surgeon's fee or the anesthesiologist's fee. You will need to get those price quotes from the doctors' office staff.

Another advantage to having your surgery in a hospital-based surgery center is that a short-stay unit or inpatient unit is available if you need it. In today's managed care environment, many operations that were formerly considered major surgeries requiring hospital admission are now being done on a same-day basis. Removal of gall bladders, (cholecystectomy); removal of the uterus (hysterectomy), and hernia repairs once required a four-to-seven day hospital stay but today patients often go home within 23 hours or less of surgery.

The evolution of new, less invasive surgical techniques
(for example, laparoscopy and endoscopy), and shorter-acting
anesthetics allows more of these formerly major procedures to be
done on a same-day or outpatient basis. However, if you experience unexpected severe discomfort and nausea – too intense to
be discharged home – you may be transferred to a *short-stay unit*
or *inpatient unit* until you recover sufficiently to go home. These
units are preferable to staying in the ambulatory surgical unit
because you will be much more comfortable in a regular hospital
bed than on the narrow, firm operating room gurney.

Office-based Surgery

In today's managed care health care market, reimbursement
to surgeons is decreasing. Some surgeons have established the
facilities, purchased the equipment, and trained the staff to perform a variety of minor surgical procedures in their offices.

Office-based surgery allows the surgeon to collect not only
their professional fee, but also some of the facility fee and supply
charges normally collected by the hospital or surgery center.
Your cost for an office-based procedure may be less than what
you would pay for the same procedure done in a surgery center.
The surgeon may charge you the same amount for his professional fee and the surgical supplies, however, his facility overhead
may be less. These savings may or may not be passed along
to you.

Office set-ups will vary with the surgeon's specialty and the
complexity of the procedures to be done in the office. Some will
limit their office procedures to simple operations that do not
require general anesthesia. Others will maintain a surgical area
much like one in an outpatient surgery setting. As with the

other "same-day" surgical sites, to have an office-based surgery you should be stable, in good health, and not require an inpatient admission.

Remember, like the free-standing sites, the quick availability of emergency services may be limited. In one case, a patient was undergoing a minor procedure in her physician's office when he inadvertently punctured her liver with an instrument. She was rushed to the local emergency department in severe shock from internal bleeding. If something serious and unexpected should happen to you, will adequate emergency care be nearby?

Also, be aware that physicians are not required to have special malpractice insurance for their office-based surgeries. This is something you might want to inquire about if you are considering an office-based procedure.

A unique advantage to office-based surgery is the privacy it affords you as a patient. Only the surgeon and his staff will know you are undergoing the procedure. Often, the office is set up with a front entrance and a separate backdoor exit. This allows you to leave after your surgery without walking through the waiting room where others can see you. Office-based surgeries are especially popular with plastic reconstructive surgeons performing cosmetic surgeries, such as eye lifts.

Hospitals

There are several types of hospitals, differentiated by a number of factors. What is sometimes confusing is that any given facility may have a combination of these factors applied to it.

The first major division is between *private* hospitals and *public* hospitals. Private hospitals are the most common type of hospitals in the United States. Most often they operate as nonprofit businesses and receive their funding from private sources (for example, local physicians or universities) or specific government funds (such as hospital bonds).

Public hospitals include those managed by a city, county, public health service, or the military. Many public hospitals provide care to society's poor. It's important to note that while these public hospitals may not have the most attractive facilities they often provide excellent care.

The second major delineation is between specialty hospitals and general hospitals. Keep in mind these may be either private or public hospitals.

Specialty Hospitals

A hospital is considered a *specialty hospital* if it provides services for only one type of patient, for instance only women or children. A facility is also considered a specialty hospital if it treats just one type of medical condition or disease such as eyes or cancer. Specialty hospitals offer expertise in a very focused area. The staff is proficient at caring for a certain population of patients or particular disease process. If your age, gender, and medical condition are within the parameters of a specialty hospital, you may want to consider seeking your care there.

General Hospitals

The majority of hospitals, whether private or public, are *general hospitals*. They treat a wider variety of patients and conditions. They usually provide medical, surgical, and diagnostic services all under one roof. However, remember these hospitals usually designate specific areas (called wards or units) for similar types of patients, essentially forming mini-specialty hospitals within themselves. For example, the heart patients are roomed in the cardiac care unit, which is separated from the children in the pediatric unit. The staff in these wards or units have considerable experience and expertise caring for the types of patients roomed in their specific area.

Osteopathic Hospitals

Osteopathic hospitals are general hospitals staffed by *Doctors of Osteopathic medicine (D.O.'s)*. The D.O.'s education, licensure, and scope of practice are very similar to that of a medical doctor. In fact, D.O.'s often practice in traditional *(allopathic)* hospitals as well as in osteopathic hospitals. The major difference between an osteopathic doctor and a medical doctor is the philosophy upon which their training is based. In addition to the more traditional medical sciences, osteopathy also teaches that a physically and psychologically intact body can defend itself against disease and heal itself. Maintaining or achieving this intact body may require the osteopathic physician to manipulate the patient's bones, joints, muscles, and other body tissues. Do not confuse an osteopathic physician – who has a medical degree – with a chiropractor who has not earned a medical degree. Chiropractors are limited to body manipulation. They do not perform surgery or provide any of the other advanced techniques physicians are licensed to do.

Veteran's Administration Hospitals

Veteran's Administration hospitals are public hospitals, but may be either specialty hospitals (for example, psychiatric hospitals) or general hospitals. They limit their patient population to members or veterans of the armed services and their dependents.

Community Hospitals

Community hospitals are private hospitals. They are predominantly general hospitals although some specialty hospitals (for example, psychiatric) do exist. They are always associated with a community or region, but not directly with a university. Depending upon whether they are in a rural or urban area, they will range in size from approximately 30 beds to several hundred beds. Community hospitals make every effort to be involved with the residents of the town in which they are located. They will often offer classes for the public on a variety of subjects, ranging from childbirth to weight control to smoking cessation. They sponsor health fairs and their staff members are encouraged to be involved with community groups and projects.

Community hospitals usually offer high-quality, fairly sophisticated medical care in a patient-focused manner. If you like personal attention, a calm atmosphere, and don't require research services or cutting-edge technology, then a community hospital may be a good choice for you.

Medical Centers

Medical centers are very large general hospitals. They may encompass several city blocks and be housed in many buildings. They offer the very latest technology and apply the latest research findings to their patient care protocols. Patients with relatively uncomplicated conditions are cared for at medical centers, but many of the patients have rare or complex conditions.

In most instances, but not all, these medical centers are affiliated with a university medical school, which means they are also teaching hospitals.

Teaching versus Non-teaching Hospitals

Quite simply, *teaching hospitals* serve as sites for educating students. The teaching hospital may be a community hospital, specialty hospital, medical center, or combination, but the common factor is that they allow students to help care for the patients. These students may be from a variety of disciplines: medicine, nursing, radiology, laboratory, physical and occupational therapy, and respiratory therapy. As a patient in a teaching hospital, there is a very good possibility you will interact with many of these students.

There are pros and cons to being a patient in a teaching hospital. On the plus side, these institutions offer the very latest technology and most recent research. The faculty are often experts in their field and have expertise in caring for a variety of complex and rare medical conditions. If you have a very complicated or uncommon condition, or if your condition requires very advanced or even experimental interventions, you may wish to choose this type of facility.

Even if your condition is common and you chose the teaching hospital for reasons other than its high-tech expertise, you will receive a considerable amount of attention as a patient. Be forewarned, not all of it may be to your liking. Medical rounds are a standard practice for teaching new doctors. This means that every day – often early in the morning and again in the evening – a covey of student doctors (medical students, interns, and residents) and their physician-instructor (attending physician) will march into your room and gather around your bed to examine you and speak to you. It can be unsettling to be awakened from a nap to find yourself surrounded by several people in white coats, all of them curious to see your incision. On the other hand, it can be very reassuring to have a great deal of attention.

In addition to teaching rounds, you may find you are visited by a succession of student doctors throughout the day. Each one may ask you the same questions and do the same examination. Student nurses may be assigned to care for you as well as students from the other disciplines. These students are closely supervised by their instructors who may also participate in your care. Some people don't mind being a teaching case and others find it too disruptive and an intolerable invasion of their privacy. You will want to carefully weigh the advantages and disadvantages of being a patient in a teaching hospital before you make your decision.

For Profit and Not-for-Profit

Hospitals are essentially businesses. They generate revenues and pay expenses just like any company. In addition, they can be operated to actually make money *(for-profit)* or to simply cover operating expenses *(not-for-profit)*. In many instances who the owner of the hospital is determines whether or not it is a for-profit or not-for profit hospital.

Consider that these hospitals can be owned by a variety of entities including, but not limited to:

- Universities
- Private corporations
- Federal, state, county, and municipal governments;
- Religious organizations
- Health maintenance organizations.

These entities may own and operate just one hospital, or they may run several hospitals. In some instances, the owner is a large corporation with multiple hospitals and other related medical facilities (such as nursing homes) located throughout the nation.

Facility Accreditation

All legitimate health care facilities must be licensed. However, not all must be accredited. Today approximately 85 percent of all hospitals in the United States have chosen to undergo the evaluation process and receive accreditation. To be accredited, the quality of health care delivered by a facility to its patients must be evaluated for compliance with nationally established standards. These standards are patient-centered performance standards against which a facility's activities and results (outcomes) are measured. Tri-annually every service and department is inspected and the quality of its care analyzed. This inspection is performed by the *Joint Commission on Accreditation of Healthcare Organizations (JCAHO)* or the American Osteopathic Association. JCAHO accreditation is required if the facility provides or participates in teaching programs or receives Medicare funding.

Managed care organizations (usually clinics and physicians' offices) are evaluated every three years against standards developed by the *National Committee for Quality Assurance (NCQA)*. The review process examines an organization's quality improvement program and looks for evidence that quality improvement activities have resulted in measurable improvement in clinical and service area performance. Accreditation allows managed care organizations to provide and participate in health care and receive payment for services rendered.

A facility's adherence to nationally recognized standards, while not a guarantee of excellent care, does imply that they strive to provide high-quality care. If a facility lacks accreditation, it is wise to ascertain why they are not accredited.

Conclusion

There are many factors to think about as you decide whether a hospital, clinic, office, or surgical center is the best surgical facility for you. Cost, where your physician is most comfortable practicing, and the availability of emergency services are three very important considerations. Also keep in mind traveling distance, the facility's reputation for quality of care, and your personal need for privacy. Each type of facility has advantages and disadvantages that only you can weigh.

CHAPTER SIX

How to Prepare for Surgery: Saving Time and Money and Avoiding Stress

Scenario

A few weeks ago you were wallpapering the bedroom and injured the muscles of your right shoulder. You had hoped that medication and physical therapy would resolve the problem. However, your shoulder continues to be extremely painful whenever you move your arm. Unfortunately, your primary care physician has diagnosed a rotator cuff tear.

Your physician referred you to a well-known orthopedic surgeon, who evaluated you yesterday. You went to the appointment prepared with several questions and, upon reviewing all the information, agreed to have an operation called a shoulder arthroscopy. Your surgery is scheduled for two weeks from today.

You feel confident that you are informed about what to expect from the surgery. You are also relieved to know that your surgeon has performed the procedure many times. Now that the difficult decision to have surgery has been made, is there anything else you should do to prepare? Yes, there certainly is.

Your decision to have an operation sets in motion a series of activities. This chapter explains why each task is important and who is responsible for its completion. By following the recommendations in this chapter, you can help prevent a last-minute delay of the operation, thereby saving time, money, and unnecessary stress.

Don't sit back and assume that everything will proceed smoothly. You want to be cooperative, but not complacent. Your responsibility is to actively participate in managing your care.

There are three main areas to be considered once you decide to have an operation.

1) *Your insurance company must authorize payment* for the operation (insurance authorization).
2) *A personalized record must be started* that contains important information about you and your health history (*preadmission paperwork*).
3) *It must be determined that you are physically healthy* enough to undergo the surgery (*preoperative physical examination*).

Elective surgical procedures are usually scheduled several weeks ahead of time in order to allow sufficient time for these important tasks to be completed. Unless you are paying cash for your operation, it's best to begin with the insurance authorization step.

Step 1: Insurance Authorization

Usually your surgeon's office staff or the hospital will call your insurance company and obtain approval for your operation. At this time, they will verify the benefits the insurance company is going to provide for your operation. However, it is a good idea for you to check directly with your insurance company to make certain you understand the amount they will pay for each portion of your hospital and physician bills.

Your insurance card – if your insurance company has provided one – contains valuable information. The front of your insurance card should contain your name, the insurance company's name, and additional information about your plan. Also on your card (perhaps on the back) you will usually find instructions about how to call for preauthorization.

Have your card, a pen, and paper ready before you place your call to the insurance representative. Be prepared to tell them the names of your primary care physician and surgeon, and their addresses and telephone numbers. Know the medical name of your operation, the approximate date of surgery, and which hospital or surgery center you and your doctor have chosen to use.

Take notes during your conversation. In addition to general notes about what services your policy covers, be certain to jot down the date, time, and full name of the person to whom you are speaking. Keep your notes in a safe place. They will serve as a reference if questions about payment for your surgery come up in the future.

Once insurance authorization has been obtained, the next step is for you to provide the hospital with information necessary for your medical record.

Step 2: Preadmission Paperwork

Completing the preadmission paperwork is often the responsibility of the admitting department in the hospital or surgery center.

An admitting department staff member will usually telephone you at home several days before your operation is scheduled. The caller will want to know your current address, telephone number, birthdate, social security number, place of employment, etc. This basic information is then used to begin your medical or hospital record.

Gathering this information early in the process allows staff to enter your data into their computer or to type the necessary papers ahead of time. On the day of your surgery, you will stop by the admitting department and your admission papers will be ready for your review and signature.

Although this makes the admission process much more efficient, not all hospitals or surgical centers use this approach. Sometimes the surgical center paperwork is less complicated than the hospital's, and you will not need to register early. If you are uncertain if your surgical site will be doing your admission paperwork ahead of time, and you would like your papers started early, call the admitting department and ask if you can give them the basic information over the telephone.

Once your insurance and admitting paperwork are in order, it's time to focus your attention on the most important aspect of your preadmission process: determining if you are able to safely undergo the surgery as scheduled.

Step 3: Presurgical Physical Examination and Tests

Today, many operations are considered "same day" surgeries. This means the patient comes into the hospital, has surgery, wakes up, and returns home all on the same day.

To streamline the process, some hospitals have established a special area for evaluating patients who are scheduled for surgery.

Names for this area may include *Preoperative Anesthesia Clinic, Preoperative Assessment Program, Preoperative Processing, Patient Assessment Unit, Preoperative Testing Unit, or Preadmission Testing Unit.*

These units are usually staffed by registered nurses, anesthesiologists, anesthesia residents, nursing aides, and clerical staff. Some units are also staffed with nurse practitioners.

Regardless of the unit's name or type of staff assigned to work in it, the purpose of this area is threefold: to assess your medical status and physical condition; to determine if laboratory tests are needed; and to perform those tests as necessary, and to provide you and your loved ones with information about your surgery and expected recovery. In a recent study of preoperative evaluation appointments, it was determined the average length for one of these appointments is about an hour and a half.

Some of your test results may take a few days to come back from the laboratory, so this preoperative evaluation is usually done several days before the scheduled surgery. If you are traveling a long distance or have a very busy schedule, arranging your surgeon's appointment and the hospital appointment on the same day will save you time and travel expenses.

Ask your surgeon what tests are planned for you, and determine if there are any documents, X-rays, or physician's orders you should hand carry to your appointment. Also ask what you should expect to happen at your preoperative assessment appointment.

During this preoperative assessment appointment you will have a physical examination. Your examiner may be a physician, an anesthesiologist, or a nurse practitioner. At this time a surgical or medical record is started. This record (or chart) will contain information on any tests that were ordered and their results when available, as well as your medical history, physical examination findings, and any other important documents.

Checking Your Vital Signs

At this time the doctor or nurse will measure your *blood pressure*, count your pulse and respirations, and take your temperature. On your chart this will often be shortened to *BP* and *TPR* or called *vital signs* ("vital" for life).

Perhaps you are wondering what blood pressure is and why it's important to measure. Blood flows through your body in a series of "pipes" called blood vessels (arteries, veins, and capillaries). It consists of nearly clear liquid (called *serum*) as well as solid particles, which include red and white blood cells. As your blood flows around, it transports food and oxygen to all of your cells while carrying waste products out for disposal through your lungs, kidneys, or liver.

Your heart is a large muscle that forces your blood through the blood vessels with a pumping action. As your heart squeezes down – or contracts – it pushes an extra measure of blood into the vessels, and this increased volume raises the pressure of the blood moving against the walls of the vessels. When the heart relaxes, the blood in the vessels is under less pressure because the extra volume isn't being forced in.

Think about running a steady stream of water through a garden hose at about half-volume, and then every five seconds cranking the faucet up to full blast for a split second before turning it down again. If you did this 70 times a minute the water would spurt or pulsate out the end of the hose 70 times a minute as the pressure changed due to the change in water volume. That's what your blood is doing inside your vessels.

When the doctor tells you about your blood pressure, you are being given information about both the highest pressure against the walls of your blood vessels during the heart's contraction, and the lowest pressure against the walls during the heart's relaxation. This is important information because it reflects how efficiently your heart is pumping blood.

This blood pressure reading consists of two numbers, the high pressure and low pressure which are written with a diagonal slash between them, and the pressure scale notation mmHg, for example: 120/80 mmHg. The higher number is called the *systolic* pressure, and the lower number the *diastolic* pressure. There is a range of what is considered normal for both the systolic and diastolic blood pressure. In a healthy adult the systolic may range from 95 to 140 and diastolic from 60 to 80 with an average of 120/80.

If the pressure is consistently abnormally high (above 140/90) the medical term is *hypertension* and if the pressure is abnormally low (below 95/60) it is termed *hypotension.*

Keep in mind, blood pressure numbers are only ranges. Your blood pressure changes throughout the day in response to your level of activity and emotions. In fact, there is a high blood pressure referred to as "white coat hypertension." It refers to the rise in blood pressure many people experience when they visit their doctor's office or the hospital.

Also, there is a good possibility your blood pressure will be elevated before your operation because of your anxiety about undergoing a surgical procedure. It would be helpful to tell your preoperative nurse what your normal blood pressure is so it can be taken into consideration during your care.

Many other things can effect the blood pressure. The following is just a partial list of what may cause changes in blood pressure:

- Blood pressure increases with excess weight
- Blood pressure is lower in newborns and highest in adults
- Blood pressure rises with stress or strong emotions
- Blood pressure may rise with extreme physical activity
- Blood pressure may change due to diseases of the circulatory system (for example, a sluggish heart will decrease blood pressure because of poor pumping action, while vessels narrowed with plaque will raise blood pressure)
- Blood pressure will drop with significant blood loss due to excessive bleeding

It's important to remember that you will not be diagnosed with high blood pressure (*hypertension*) unless after several readings on different days you consistently have a blood pressure reading higher than the normal range for your age and condition.

If you have been diagnosed with high blood pressure (or, in medical terms *chronic hypertension*) there are many medications available that help control your blood pressure and maintain it at a safe level. If your physician has prescribed high blood pressure medication for you, it's very important that you follow the directions for its use in order to prevent complications or illness. And don't forget to list it with your medications to be discussed with your preoperative examiner.

Your *body temperature* will also be measured prior to surgery. Usually, this is done with a thermometer placed under your tongue or against your ear for a short time. Thermometers vary, so carefully follow the nurse's instructions.

The normal range of the human body's internal temperature (measured in your mouth) is 97.7°–99.5° Farenheit (F), or

36.5°–37.5° Centigrade (C). This is the very narrow range allowable if your body is to function correctly. A temperature that varies only 4 degrees either above or below normal can result in convulsions.

An elevated temperature may be caused by several conditions. The most frequent reason for a higher than normal temperature is some type of infection: for example, the flu, strep throat, or postoperative infection. Temperature may also rise if there is a problem with the brain, such as swelling. Sometimes the body's thermostat, which is located within the brain, malfunctions and results in a temperature increase. And finally, if a person is exposed to excessively high heat — perhaps walking through the desert or playing tennis on an especially hot and humid day — it can cause a dangerous rise in body temperature.

If you have an elevated temperature prior to surgery, your physician will want to postpone your operation until a reason can be evaluated. Your doctor will also want you to feel better before going into surgery.

The rate, volume, and rhythm of your heartbeat *(pulse)* will be assessed as well as the rate and pattern of your breaths *(respirations)*.

Preoperative Tests

Laboratory tests, chest X-rays, and electrocardiograms (EKG/ECG) may also be part of this preoperative examination. Each state has specific requirements for preoperative patient preparation. Some states require basic laboratory tests such as urine analysis, complete blood cell count, or measurements of red blood cell volume (hematocrit) and the oxygen carrying capacity of red blood cells (hemoglobin). Patients with special medical problems (or over 40 years of age) often are required to have an EKG (tracing of their heart's electrical activity) and/or a chest X-ray. Other states leave it up to the surgeon to decide which tests are necessary.

Let's briefly discuss these basic tests so you are informed about what will be happening to you.

Laboratory Tests

A urine analysis (*urinalysis*) used to be a routine test performed on every surgical patient. Today, that practice varies greatly. Don't be overly concerned if your physician does not order a urine test. A urinalysis is actually several tests done on one sample of urine you provide. Instructions for obtaining a urine sample are usually posted in the bathroom of the clinic or laboratory. If they aren't, ask someone how to clean yourself and correctly catch some urine into the small plastic cup they have given you.

Your urine will be tested for the presence of blood cells (which may indicate an infection), sugar (which may indicate diabetes), proteins (which may indicate kidney disease) as well as its specific gravity (which measures your body's fluid concentration).

If your physician orders a complete blood count, hemoglobin or hematocrit, blood will be drawn from your arm or from a pin prick in your finger.

The technician may fill several small glass tubes with blood. Some tests require that specific tubes be used in order to correctly preserve the blood specimen. It may look like they are taking a lot of blood, but each tube only holds about a teaspoonful (and you have several quarts of blood in your body). These blood tests help determine if you are physically stable enough to have surgery.

Chest X-rays

Chest X-rays are often ordered prior to surgery. Physicians will check your X-ray to make certain your lungs are healthy and have no fluid or infection in them. This ensures that your post-operative recovery is not complicated by an already existing lung problem that can lead to pneumonia.

Chest X-rays are painless although you may find the X-ray room chilly. You will be dressed in a hospital gown, and then asked to either lie on a hard table or to stand in front of a flat-surfaced machine. The technician will slide a large metal frame containing X-ray film into a slot in the table or wall behind you.

Follow the technician's instructions when you are asked to breathe deeply or hold your breath, so that your picture is sharp and focused. You may hear a loud click, but there will be no discomfort.

For many years, all of the preoperative tests we have discussed were considered necessary for evaluating a patient's ability to safely undergo surgery. In today's health care market, managed care's increasing pressure for cost-effective utilization of services means tests are ordered only if there is reason to believe the patient may not be physically stable enough for surgery, or if the test is required by the hospital or state regulations.

Electrocardiogram (EKG/ECG)

If you are scheduled for an EKG you should know it is a painless test that is used to evaluate the efficiency of your heart.

Each heartbeat mechanically pushes blood — carrying vital oxygen, food, and waste products — through your arteries and veins to every cell in your body. Each heart beat also creates electrical energy that you never feel.

Using specialized equipment, this electrical energy can be mapped out onto a piece of graph paper. By studying the graph made by your heartbeat, the doctor can determine if your heart is strong enough to withstand anesthesia and surgery. If an abnormality is detected, you may require additional testing, or your surgery may be delayed until your heart problem is resolved.

What happens during the EKG? The technician will wheel a small machine beside your bed and painlessly attach it to your body. Depending upon the type of EKG machine, this may mean three long wires that have small, round, paper or foam disks on their ends will be placed on your chest and leg. These disks will be sticky – like an adhesive Band-Aid – and may have a small glob of clear jelly in their center. The disks are called electrodes or monitor leads. The jelly (which sometimes feels wet or cold) helps the machine pick up the electrical impulses your heart generates.

The technician will start running the graph paper through the machine and in some instances a pen will bounce up and down, tracing a wavy line. You may be able to hear the whir of the moving paper and the scratching noise of the pen as it records your heartbeat, but you will not feel any discomfort. Some machines are silent. The technician may make notations on the paper. This is normal.

After a minute or two, the EKG is complete. The electrodes are no longer needed, and unless you are especially hairy, their removal is also painless. Ask for a tissue to remove any residual jelly.

Medical History Questionnaire

Many hospitals make this whole preadmission physical evaluation process easier and quicker by asking you to fill out a medical history questionnaire. This completed questionnaire is then carefully reviewed by the physician or nurse doing your physical examination.

It is very important that you answer each question as completely and as honestly as possible. Based upon the information you provide and the results of your physical examination, your health status is evaluated in relationship to your ability to undergo surgery and anesthesia. Your examiner will decide if you need additional tests and will discuss this with you.

The Three Critical Questions

All of the questions you will be asked are important. However, there are three that are critically important. They are:

- "Have you had any previous surgeries and did you experience any problems or complications with these operations?"
- "What medications are you currently taking?"
- "Do you have any allergies?"

Previous Surgeries

Information about previous surgeries is important because it tells the examiner about your ability to tolerate anesthesia and avoid postoperative complications. Briefly tell the person examining you about your past operations. Was your operation or were your operations successful? Did you wake up quickly and without severe nausea or headache? How would you describe your postoperative pain? Did you recover quickly? Did your wound heal quickly? Did you have any postoperative problems such as bleeding, pneumonia, or infection?

Medications

It's very helpful for you to bring a list of all the medications you are currently taking to your preoperative appointment.

Write down the name of each drug; the strength or dose (usually noted as milligrams or mgs or cc's); how often you take it; when you took your last dose; and why you are taking it. We have provided a form for you to photocopy and use at the end of Chapter 12.

Don't forget about any over-the-counter medications you may be taking. Even though they do not require a doctor's prescription to buy, over-the-counter medications can still be potent drugs. Something as common as aspirin, which is often an ingredient in cold medicines, can interfere with your blood clotting mechanism and make it more difficult to stop bleeding.

Depending upon your medications and their effect, you may be asked to temporarily stop taking certain drugs or to change the amount you take. Write down next to each medication on your list what the new instructions are for its use during your preoperative period.

If you use illicit or "recreational" drugs, now is the time to discuss this with your physician. He or she will keep this information confidential.

Allergies

The only way to know if you are allergic to a medication is if you have taken it previously and it caused an unexpected and undesired reaction in your body. This type of reaction is called an allergic reaction because your body reacted to the chemicals in the medication as though they were harmful foreign matter.

These abnormal or allergic reactions can take several forms. Sometimes they appear as a skin rash or "hives." Other times they cause severe nausea, wheezing, and facial swelling. Additionally, some drugs can cause feelings of restlessness, nervousness, and hyperactivity, or extreme fatigue and listlessness. The most severe form of an allergic reaction is called *anaphylactic shock*. This is an extremely serious and potentially life threatening reaction which includes loss of consciousness, difficulty breathing, and extremely low blood pressure.

If you have ever taken any medication (pills, liquid, ointment, inhaler, or powder) or used any products (for example, bandages, tape, sutures, iodine soap) and experienced an unexpected or unpleasant reaction, it's critical that you alert the person doing your examination. Tell them exactly what drug or product you reacted to and specifically what happened when you took it. Did you have nausea? A skin rash? Wheezing? Dizziness? Nervousness or extreme tiredness?

Allergic reactions may tend to get worse with each episode. Also, many drugs are chemically related, so if you are allergic to one you may be allergic to another in the same family. Providing your allergy information will assist the health care professional in anticipating any reaction you might have to other drugs. The doctor will not prescribe any medications or use any products you are known to be allergic to. You can help monitor your medications by asking everyone who gives you medication for the name of the medication and why they are giving it to you.

During the preoperative assessment, you should also discuss blood products if your surgery will require you to receive blood replacement. This is something you have already discussed with your surgeon, but the donation details may not have been worked out.

If you will lose enough blood during your operation to require a blood transfusion there are several options to consider.

The safest type of blood replacement is to receive your own blood (self-donation) because it is a perfect match and you know your medical history. Hospitals have made it very convenient for people to donate their own blood and store it in the blood bank for use during their surgery. However, there needs to be a certain time interval (usually a few weeks) between the donations and the surgery for this choice to be available to you.

The next safest choice is to receive blood from a known donor; for example a spouse, child, relative, or close friend. Be aware that the donor's blood type and your blood type must match in order for this option to work. There are four major blood types: A, B, AB, and O. Also, there is a factor called the Rh factor which is either present (positive) or absent (negative).

Ideally, these factors and several additional minor factors must match in order to avoid a very serious and potentially fatal reaction. As with self-donation, there is a certain time that must be allowed between the blood donation and the surgery.

Finally, if the options of self-donation or use of a known donor are not available to you, you will receive carefully matched blood from the hospital blood bank. Please be assured that you need not fear contracting diseases from blood supplied by the hospital blood bank. The hospitals perform many tests on all the blood in their bank and the risk of catching any disease is minuscule.

Education

The final component of your preoperative appointment may be education about your upcoming surgery. It's a good idea to take notes and/or to bring a family member or friend who will be involved with your postoperative care.

A nurse will instruct you in the proper procedures for maintaining wellness immediately after your operation. You will be given instruction about deep breathing and coughing exercises to keep your lungs clear. You may also be given information about your expected level of activity and any anticipated need for pain medication. We discuss these subjects in Chapter 11.

This is an excellent opportunity for both you and a significant other to gather additional information about what is going to happen to your body as a result of the surgery and what your expected recovery will be like. Some of these educational programs will include discussion with physical therapists if you will require rehabilitation, or a case manager if you will require hospitalization.

CHAPTER SEVEN

Legal Considerations

Scenario

You're scheduled for surgery in a few days and your friend Eleanor telephones to reassure you. In the course of your conversation she tells you "Get ready to sign a lot of paperwork. I signed my name to at least four forms, almost as many as when I bought my house!" You begin to worry. What forms are you going to be requested to sign and why? Should you be concerned about legal issues? What rights do you have?

Our health care system recognizes *patient autonomy*. This means that you, as a patient, have the right to independence, freedom, and self-determination. This autonomy guarantees you the right to consent to or refuse treatment and means that health care providers are legally and ethically obligated to conform to what is called the informed consent process.

The Patient Bill of Rights

In addition, a *Patient Bill of Rights* has been written and approved by national and statewide hospital organizations, medical societies, nursing organizations, and other groups of health professionals. The Patient Bill of Rights describes the rights you are entitled to when receiving health care services. These rights include:

- Care given without regard to race, sex, ethnicity, religion, or source of payment
- Consideration and respect
- Information about the health care providers, the illness, treatment and alternatives, prognosis, and risks of treatment
- Informed consent or refusal
- Protection of privacy and confidentiality
- Reasonable responses to any reasonable requests
- The right to leave the hospital against medical advice
- The right to be informed about any part of health care that is research, as well as the right to refuse to participate in research
- Information about health care requirements at home
- The right to a full examination and explanation of the hospital bill
- The right to know hospital rules and regulations that affect patient conduct such as visiting limitations, smoking prohibitions, etc.
- The extension of the Bill of Rights to the person who has legal responsibility for making health care decisions

In 1990, federal legislation called the *Patient Self-Determination Act* was also passed requiring all hospitals and health care agencies receiving Medicaid or Medicare funds to advise patients about their right to consent to and/or refuse treatment and about the availability of advance directives such as a living will or durable power of attorney. We will discuss advance directives later in this chapter.

Informed Consent

First let's consider the informed consent process. The informed consent process requires that the person performing your treatment or operation be legally and ethically responsible for providing you with complete information about your procedure and also be responsible for obtaining your consent to perform the procedure on you.

Simply stated, your surgeon and anesthesiologist must give you all of the facts regarding your case and, after having completely informed you to your satisfaction, must get your permission to proceed with your operation. Because you only give your consent after you are fully informed about your situation, this is referred to as informed consent.

What information should you be provided with in order to make an informed decision? According to the Patient Bill of Rights, which is recognized in all states, and by state law in some states, you are entitled to know the following:

- The name of the physician who has primary responsibility for coordinating your care, and the names and roles of any other physicians and non-physicians who will be participating in your care
- The nature of your illness or health problem; the treatment or procedures indicated; the prospects for your recovery
- The risks, complications, and expected benefits or effects of the treatment
- Any alternatives to treatment and their risks or benefits

This final right is especially important in a managed care environment. Remember, there are several factors which may discourage your HMO physician from discussing more expensive treatment alternatives with you. First, in a *capitated system* your primary care physician is compensated with a fixed amount of money for your care. He or she is "at risk" financially if more money is spent caring for you than the stipend covers. Second, HMOs monitor the amount of money their network physicians spend on patient care. A physician who is perceived to be spending more than the normal amount of money may be removed from the network. Third, HMOs may stipulate in their contracts with physicians that if they speak negatively against the HMO, challenge HMO decisions about treatment approvals, or complain about the HMO, they may be removed from the network panel.

The information in the Patient's Bill of Rights should be complete and must be provided in words you can understand. The names and descriptions of procedures should be stated in terms that are commonly used and abbreviations should be avoided. For example, a *bilateral salpingo-oophorectomy (BSO)* should be described as "removal of the ovaries and Fallopian tubes which are necessary for pregnancy."

Exactly how detailed should the information be and what risks should be discussed? Your physician is legally required to provide the information which a reasonable person in your position would need to know in order to consent to or refuse treatment. If the patient has special circumstances and concerns (for example, a professional singer who may be worried about vocal cord damage during an operation to remove abnormal growths on the vocal cords) any special concerns should be discussed.

If you know there is specific information about your procedure that's very important for you to have in order to make your decision to consent or refuse, you should ask for that information directly. For instance, if you're worried about an unsightly scar forming and would refuse the operation even if there is only a slight chance of significant scarring, you should ask about the risk of getting an unsightly scar.

Giving care or performing procedures without your informed consent is a legal offense called *battery*. Battery is defined as offensive or injurious physical contact; however your injury does not need to have resulted from the physical contact. It is enough that you did not consent to the physical contact.

Battery is a civil offense resulting in money damages paid to the patient. If a health care provider is found guilty of battery, he or she may be subjected to professional discipline such as suspension or revocation of a professional license and loss of privileges to provide specific types of health care.

In addition, failure to provide informed consent associated with injury to the patient may be part of the evidence showing professional malpractice. All of these consequences are dependent upon patients who are informed of their rights and willing to make complaints when those rights are ignored.

When you are having surgery, the persons responsible for carrying out your informed consent process are your surgeon and your anesthesiologist. While these people are responsible for obtaining your consent and permission, the required information may be provided via other sources such as pamphlets, videotapes and discussion with patient educators and nurses. It's important to understand that, regardless of the methods used to give you the information, the only person accountable for the accuracy of that information is the person performing the procedure.

If you're not satisfied with the information provided in the pamphlets, videos, or discussions with educators, or if you obtain information from these other sources which makes you reconsider a decision to consent to a procedure, you should state you are considering refusing the operation and ask to speak to the responsible physician. You're always entitled to an informative interview with the treating physician in order to obtain additional information or have questions answered about what will be done during the procedure and the risks involved.

As a competent adult, you're entitled to consent to, or refuse, your treatment. To be considered competent you must be aware of who you are, where you are, and be capable of understanding the nature and consequences of what you are being asked to consent to. You are assumed to be competent unless there is evidence to the contrary and a determination of incompetency has been made by the court system. In this instance, the court will appoint a guardian or conservator who is legally entitled to all of the same rights as the patient in regard to informed consent.

In some other countries, a husband is required to consent or refuse treatment for his wife. In this country only you, as a competent adult, can consent to or refuse treatment for yourself. As long as you are competent, your consent or refusal stands, even if your husband or another family member disagrees with your decision.

An adult is defined as a person eighteen years of age or older. Children (minors) must obtain the consent of their parents or legal guardians for most treatments or procedures. There are some exceptions to this rule, that vary from state to state, regarding a minor's right to consent to treatment for pregnancy or sexually related problems. When a parent or guardian is not available for consent, and the health problem is life-threatening, the health care provider may assume that consent is implied and proceed with the procedure.

What happens in an emergency when you may be temporarily incompetent (for example, unconscious after an accident)? The physician treating you, or the hospital, may use what is called *implied consent*. Implied consent means that it is inferred that you consent to whatever treatment is necessary to save your life and preserve your health.

The physician responsible for treating you may go ahead and initiate the emergency procedures indicated by your condition. In such a situation, you may actually receive treatment that you would have refused had you been competent. After you regain consciousness and become competent, implied consent no longer applies and your consent or refusal must be obtained for any further treatments.

Several of the forms you will be asked to sign concern legal issues surrounding informed consent. The day of your surgery, when you are nervous, thirsty, and wishing everything was over, may not be the best time to try to concentrate on the small print at the bottom of the pages.

You are entitled to review these documents in advance and to question anything that's unclear to you. If you prefer to read the forms prior to the day of surgery, call the admitting department and request the forms be sent to you. If you have questions, the admitting personnel will be able to answer most of them or will refer you to an administrator or your physician for more detailed answers.

The forms should be written in plain language using terms you can understand. You are entitled to an interpreter if English is not your primary language and you prefer to discuss such important matters in your native tongue. We advise you to use a specially trained interpreter provided by the hospital or surgical center rather than a family member or friend. This is simply

because your family member or friend may not be familiar
with the medical terms and may be unable to make an accurate
translation.

The Forms

The two important forms you will always encounter are the
admission consent form and the procedure consent form. In
addition, you may ask to see two additional legal documents
called advance directives. These *advance directives* are commonly
referred to as a *living will* and a *durable power of attorney* form.

The admission form generally states that you, as the patient,
voluntarily consent to be admitted to the hospital or surgical
center, that you agree to receive care from the facility's personnel, accept financial responsibility for services provided, and will
comply with any conflict resolution procedures or arbitration the
facility may require in the event of a dispute.

It's important to understand this admission consent form
may be consented to in part and refused in part. In other words,
you do not have to agree to the entire contents of the form.
Some patients may refuse the services of certain categories of
facility personnel such as students, interns, or residents. Refusal
of services is always the right of the patient and the facility has
an ethical obligation to make reasonable responses to reasonable
requests. This means they must do what is reasonable to comply
with your request.

If you know you prefer to refuse certain elements of the
admission consent, it's best to discuss these issues with your
physician in advance so the consequences of your refusal can
be discussed.

In some situations, the admission form may contain statements about the patient agreeing not to sue or agreeing to com-

ply with the facility's *arbitration* procedures. No one can be compelled to waive their legal right to appear in a court of law in order to obtain health care services. Statements about agreeing not to sue are generally not enforced by the courts, even when the patient voluntarily signs them as part of a larger document to obtain health care.

Agreeing to comply with arbitration means that before filing a law suit, the patient agrees to have a neutral group review their claim and decide whether or not it has merit and what damages, if any, are fair. If you agree to arbitration, you must go through the arbitration process before filing a law suit. If you are unhappy with the results of the arbitration process, you may proceed with a law suit after arbitration is completed.

The second form, the informed consent for the procedure, is your permission for the procedure(s) or operation(s) to be done to you. If anesthesia is required, you will also be asked to give permission for the administration of anesthesia. Usually there is a separate form for each procedure to be done. While some of these consents may be given orally, consent for surgery is usually given in writing. There will be a place for your signature which must be written or printed by you. Your full legal signature must be used. Someone must witness you signing the forms. This witness is not verifying that the informed consent process was legally and ethically performed, but rather simply verifying it truly is your signature on the form. Usually this witness is the admitting clerk or nurse.

Patients may become confused about who is responsible for the informed consent process because it is a nurse or admitting clerk rather than the physician who asks them to sign the actual form. Keep in mind, the role of the hospital staff is to verify that the informed consent process has been carried out by your physician and to be certain the signed forms are included in your patient record.

The staff will ask you if you have spoken with your physician about the surgery and then will ask you to sign the appropriate forms. If you have not spoken to your physician, or if your information was unsatisfactory, or you have unanswered questions, you should delay signing the form until you can speak to your physician. The staff cannot answer questions about the procedure. They will contact and inform your physician that your consent has not been obtained and is dependent upon your receiving additional information from the physician.

If the only available version of the forms is in English and the consent is obtained in a different language, the services of an interpreter should be obtained to translate the form and obtain the patient's signature. The form should indicate an interpreter was used and the interpreter should sign as well.

These forms should always have the accurate time and date on them. All language should be common usage and no abbreviations should be used. The physician's name and title should be completely spelled out so it is clear who is the responsible party. If two physicians have the same name (for example father and son), correct identifying information should be included.

The name of the procedure (operation) should be in common terms and completely spelled out. It is important to note that not all of the treatments, alternatives and risks may be listed or described. These consent forms only document that the consent process, which should have included an opportunity for an informative discussion, answers to questions and a discussion of the risks, was completed. The forms do not describe the exact contents of the discussion nor do they describe the process itself.

Signing an informed consent document does not bind you forever. You may change your mind and revoke your consent at any time, whether it's one second or several hours after signing your name. It's important to recognize that the amount of time between consent and refusal is irrelevant. Even in the rare situation when the patient signs the consent and then immediately changes his or her mind and refuses, their refusal stands. There is no point in time when a consent cannot be revoked. The facility and physicians are legally required to comply with your refusal, no matter what the consequences. Your refusal may be verbal and may be communicated to any member of the staff. Anyone who hears a patient refusal is obligated to inform the responsible physician that the signed consent is not valid.

One of the most common fears for those about to have surgery is the fear of a disaster or terrible accident occuring during the procedure. What will happen if you become permanently unconscious or unable to make decisions (incompetent)?

Advance Directives

There are two legal documents which will allow you to make a decision to consent or refuse treatment in advance. These are called advance directives and include a living will and a durable power of attorney.

Many states have recognized the right of persons to control decisions about life-saving or life-prolonging treatment in advance, anticipating that they might be rendered unable to make decisions at the time the treatment is ordered. If the patient has a living will, it will state specifically which life-sustaining measures he permits or refuses.

The living will allows a person who may develop a terminal illness or a permanent unconscious/vegetative state that makes it impossible for them to make decisions about their care, to indicate in advance what life-sustaining measures he or she agrees to or refuses. (A terminal illness is defined as an illness which is likely to result in death within a relatively short amount of time.)

When a patient develops a terminal illness or a permanent vegetative state that makes it impossible for them to make decisions about their care, two physicians must certify the person is unable to make decisions for themselves. At this point, a competency proceeding will be conducted in a court of law to identify a guardian for the patient. This guardian will then consent or refuse the patient's treatment. If a living will exists, the terms of the living will apply.

The signing of a living will must be witnessed by two persons, at least one of whom has no expectation of inheritance from the person making the will. Health care providers or employees (i.e., nurses) of health care agencies where the patient is hospitalized may not witness the will.

It's important to understand that a living will has nothing to do with the type of will that leaves property to a person's heirs after death. A living will is effective while the person is still alive, hence the term "living will." A will that leaves property is not effective — or for that matter even opened and read — until the person has died. It's important that statements about life-sustaining treatments not be put in the property will, which is never opened until after death.

Durable power of attorney is a legal document in which a competent adult gives to another competent adult the right to make his or her health care decisions, including the refusal of life-sustaining treatments, should the person writing the durable power of attorney document become unable to make decisions for him or herself. This document must also be witnessed by two people. The same restrictions for heirs, health care providers, and employees of the hospital apply.

Note the difference between a living will and a durable power of attorney document. A living will allows the person writing the will to make decisions about personal health care in advance. A durable power of attorney document allows someone else to make decisions when the person writing the document is no longer capable of making decisions.

A durable power of attorney document is more flexible than a living will because it is difficult for someone writing a living will to anticipate all the decisions that might be required in the course of their treatment. However, a durable power of attorney document relies on trust that the person making decisions will make the same decisions as the person writing the document.

These advance directives are a very powerful way for persons to control decisions about saving or sustaining their lives when they are unable to make decisions for themselves. It is best if you think carefully about these documents and complete them in advance. There are some important things to remember in order for these documents to be effective.

Before the Documents Take Effect

The documents must be written correctly. There is legal language that should be included in the document. Forms are available in the hospital and many office supply stores or bookstores that are correctly worded and require only that you fill in the blanks. It's best to use a pre-printed form such as those distributed by the medical association or hospital association.

The documents must be signed by you, the person they are intended for, and the act of signing must be witnessed by two persons, not health care providers or heirs. If the documents are not properly witnessed, they will not be enforced. Too often people put off writing them until their final minutes when they are very ill and only family members and hospital staff are available to witness the signing. As we discussed earlier in this chapter, these people may not serve as witnesses in this situation.

The documents are not effective if no one knows about them. You may be unconscious when the documents are needed. Originals should be kept by the person most likely to be with you in the hospital. At the time of admission, the original documents should be given to the admitting clerk to include in the hospital chart. Only the original documents will be enforced.

It's helpful to tell the responsible physician that there are advance directives, but it's not foolproof. Often the physician who admits the patient to the hospital turns patient care responsibilities over to medical specialists as the patient becomes sicker and develops complications. The original physician who was notified may not be involved in the patient's care when the documents are needed. Your or your family should remind each physician that advance directives have been signed.

In the case of durable power of attorney, it's very important to have a serious discussion with the person being designated to make your health care decisions. It's important for you to inform this person about what treatments you want to refuse so they will make the same decision you would if you were capable of making your own decisions. It's also important to remember that those closest to you, your spouse or children, may have the most difficulty making decisions that become associated with your death.

All advance directives can be revoked immediately and at any time by you, the person who wrote them.

In some circumstances, the courts have enforced prior patient statements about their desires for treatment decisions, even when the legal documents have not been signed.

Therefore, it is critically important for you to discuss your feelings and preferences with someone close to you even when you have not completed legal documents. Completion of legal documents will certainly strengthen the likelihood that your wishes will be enforced, but even oral statements may help your preferences be met.

Organ Donation

Another area where it is extremely important to keep family members and friends informed about your preferences concerns organ donation. Your family members or significant others will often be asked to consider donation of your organs very close to the time of death. If you have designated yourself as a donor with an attachment to your driver's license or discussed your preferences at the time of admission and documented them in the hospital consent form, your preferences will be quietly followed and your loved ones will be spared the pain and stress of making the decision for you. Organs may not be donated without the express consent of the patient or legally responsible family member.

The "Do Not Resuscitate" Order

One other legal consideration is that of a *do not resuscitate* order. This is not an issue of informed consent or refusal made by the patient. Instead, it is an order that comes from the physician directing the hospital and nursing staff about what should be done in the event the patient stops breathing and/or their heart stops beating. When this happens, and there is a "do not resuscitate" order, the staff will not make any attempts to restore breathing or a heart beat. No stimulating medications will be given and no life-support measures will be started.

A physician will only write an order not to resuscitate when the patient and the family have agreed that it's the best course of action. It's necessary for the physician to write and sign such an order on the patient's chart in order to prevent resuscitative efforts.

CHAPTER EIGHT

An Update on Anesthesia: Improved, Safer Techniques

Scenario

Your last surgery was a tonsillectomy when you were a child. Although your memories have faded, you can still recall the frightening, suffocating sensation you had when instructed to inhale strange smelling ether through a rubber mask placed over your nose and mouth. Nor have you forgotten how the promises of "all the ice cream you can eat" were negated by the waves of nausea you felt upon awakening. Do you have to worry about having this unpleasant anesthetic experience again with the surgery you have recently scheduled? Be assured, you do not.

Unfortunately, for many people the thought of receiving an anesthetic still conjures up the terrible memories of ether anesthetic. This is despite the fact that anesthetic agents, and the techniques for administering them, have markedly improved. Not only is the experience of general anesthesia much less unpleasant, but it is also far safer than ever before. In fact, the malpractice insurance carriers now consider anesthesiologists to be a lower malpractice risk than they were 10 years ago because of the lower incidence of anesthetic-related problems.

Anesthesiologists have done little to educate the public or their colleagues in the health professions about the improvements in anesthesia. What follows is a discussion of what you, as the patient, can expect from your anesthetic experience.

The Anesthesiologist

Your surgeon will discuss your upcoming operation in detail with you. She will review the actual procedure, the relative risks and benefits of the proposed procedure, and what you can expect postoperatively. She may also briefly describe various anesthetic options. However, it is the anesthesiologist who is best qualified to determine what the most appropriate anesthetic option should be, based upon the planned surgical procedure and your overall health.

You should consider your anesthesiologist as your "internist" in the operating room. He or she is the person who will not only provide your anesthesia, but will also be in charge of maintaining all your bodily functions at a normal level during the surgery. This is a demanding role and requires a great deal of expertise.

The anesthesiologist has completed a long period of training before going into practice. This training includes: undergraduate school (usually four years of college); four years of medical school; one year of internship; and three-to-four years of residency specializing in anesthesia. The fourth year of residency training may be in an anesthesia subspecialty, such as cardiac, pediatric, or obstetrical anesthesia; pain management; or critical care.

After the completion of a residency, the anesthesiologist must pass a rigorous written and oral examination given by the American Board of Anesthesiology in order to become a board certified anesthesiologist. The anesthesiologist may then practice anesthesia as a professor in an academic institution (for example, training residents) or as a private practitioner.

He or she may also practice in a hospital with nurse anesthetists. These nurses are registered nurses who have had additional training in anesthesia. They provide anesthesia to patients under the direct supervision of a physician anesthesiologist.

Questions you should ask about the qualifications of your anesthesia provider include:

1. Is the anesthesiologist board certified?
2. How many years has this person practiced anesthesia?
3. How familiar is he or she with your surgeon and your type of surgery?
4. If an anesthesia resident trainee will be involved in your anesthesia care, how will they be supervised?

Preoperative Interview

You will have a very important preoperative interview with your anesthesiologist before your scheduled surgery. This may take place a few days before your operation, by telephone the night before surgery, or in the preoperative area on the day of surgery.

At this time the anesthesiologist will review with you your general medical history, the medications you take on a regular basis, your drug allergies and your previous surgical or anesthetic experiences, and any possible complications you might have experienced in the past. You have already told this information to a number of health care professionals; however, you may find that you have to repeat some of the same information for the anesthesiologist. You should always answer honestly and to the best of your ability.

During this discussion the anesthesiologist will answer your questions and help allay your fears about the upcoming anesthetic. None of your questions will be considered too minor to answer. Consider writing down all of your questions before the interview to ensure that all of your concerns are addressed.

After discussing your medical history with you, the anesthesiologist will review the results of your preoperative tests and at
some point perform a brief physical examination. Evaluating all
of this data will help the anesthesiologist decide not only if you
are ready for surgery and anesthesia, but also what type of anesthetic technique and monitoring will be best for you.

The decision about the type of anesthetic and how it will be
administered will rest with you and your anesthesiologist. There
are many factors which contribute to the selection of one anesthetic plan over another. Some of the variables include the type
of surgical procedure; the surgical site; your predisposing medical
conditions; the length of time required for the surgery; and the
expected discharge and recovery plan. Remember, the anesthesiologist is an expert consultant who is highly qualified to design a
safe and effective anesthetic plan for you.

Regardless of the anesthetic treatment plan you and your
anesthesiologist have agreed upon, you can expect to have an
I.V. or *intravenous line* started. As discussed earlier, this is plastic
tubing attached to a needle that is inserted into the middle of
one of your veins. Sterile solution is then run through the tubing
and into your vein. This establishes immediate access to your
bloodstream so that medications can be injected repeatedly into
the solution or tubing rather than repeatedly into your arm.
Medications administered in this way have a very fast action and
the anesthesiologist is able to carefully control the drug's effect.

Your anesthesiologist will start your I.V. with minimal discomfort. Usually a small amount of local anesthetic or numbing
medicine will be injected into the site with a very tiny needle
before the larger "I.V." needle is inserted. This I.V. will remain
in place until just before your discharge from the hospital.
There is seldom any discomfort when the I.V. is removed.

In addition to planning your anesthetic treatment, your anesthesiologist will stay next to you and constantly monitor you while you are in the operating room. Your anesthesia will be administered in carefully calculated increments, customized for you, so you are always comfortable or asleep. The anesthetic treatment is much too complicated for the anesthesiologist to simply give you a dose of anesthetic and then leave you alone.

Generally, it is the anesthesiologist who makes the final decision as to whether you are in the best physical and medical condition to undergo anesthesia and surgery at this time. Your internist and surgeon have both participated in evaluating you for surgery, but they rely on the anesthesiologist's medical judgment, knowledge of the surgery, and anesthesia expertise to make the final decision about proceeding.

There are several reasons your scheduled surgery may be postponed at the last minute. This can be very frustrating, but remember it is in your best interest. You will have been instructed to have nothing to eat or drink for at least eight hours before your operation is scheduled to begin. This is meant as a safety precaution. When under anesthesia, the body's normal reflexes that protect the airway from stomach contents are suppressed. An empty stomach prevents the possibility of gastric (stomach) contents being aspirated (vomited and inhaled) into your lungs as you undergo your anesthetic. If you have had anything to eat or drink too close to the time of surgery, your operation may be rescheduled.

Your operation will also be rescheduled for another day if you have a cold and cough at the time of surgery. This is a safety precaution, meant to prevent postoperative respiratory complications. If any of your laboratory test results were initially abnormal, the anesthesiologist may request a repeat test on the day of your surgery to see if your results have returned to a normal range. This will only be necessary if the abnormal test affects the anesthetic or surgical plan. If any of your vital signs are different from your normal baseline (for example, your blood pressure is unusually high, your heartbeat is newly irregular, or you have a fever) that may also delay your surgery.

Your surgery will only be postponed if, after very careful evaluation, your anesthesiologist and surgeon determine that the risk of surgery and anesthesia outweighs the benefits at this point in time.

Monitoring in the Operating Room

The emotional stress of surgery, the anesthetic medications, the surgical procedure itself, and many other factors can alter your normal physiological state during surgery. Therefore, it is critical that your anesthesiologist constantly monitor your vital signs.

The American Society of Anesthesiologists and state law have established minimal monitoring guidelines. You can expect that, at minimum, your blood pressure, heart rate and rhythm, respiratory pattern, and the amount of oxygen in your blood will be constantly evaluated.

The most common equipment used for this monitoring is termed *non-invasive*, which means it simply rests on the outside of your body. It includes a blood pressure cuff, an EKG monitor, a stethoscope on your chest, and a *pulse oximeter*. The latter is a small Band Aid-like strip or soft clip that gently fastens onto a fingertip. Utilizing infrared spectrometry, it keeps track of your blood oxygen level. This monitor, developed within the past 15 years, has revolutionized safety in anesthesia. It is exquisitely sensitive to small changes in the level of oxygen in your blood so that early warning of any problems can be immediately recognized and treated before escalating into potentially more serious problems.

Occasionally, either because of the complexity of the surgical procedure or your particular medical condition, more extensive monitoring will be necessary to ensure the safest surgical, anesthetic, and postoperative course for you. This additional monitoring may require what is called "invasive" monitoring or equipment that requires some form of insertion into the body. Examples include sophisticated *intravenous lines, intra-arterial lines,* and special *echocardiographic* or *electroencephalographic* monitors. The necessity of these monitoring devices will be determined by your anesthesiologist in conjunction with your surgeon.

Generally, it is the anesthesiologist who is in charge of placing these special monitors, interpreting the information they provide, and acting on this information. As with your I.V. insertion, your anesthesiologist will place these devices with minimal discomfort.

Surgery Under Local Anesthesia: No Anesthesiologist Present

In some instances, your surgery can be performed with only a *local anesthetic.* The term local anesthetic refers to the injection of numbing medications into only the part of your body that is to be operated upon, similar to when your dentist injects Novocain into your jaw during dental procedures. The anesthetic medications used are often a mixture of drugs, such as adrenaline plus additional agents, which take effect quickly, and also others that last a long time. As stated earlier, during the surgery you will be aware of touch and pressure, but you should not feel sharp pain. More local anesthesia will be injected if you feel sharp pain.

Local anesthesia can be used for certain surgeries which are limited in their complexity and duration. If you are having this type of anesthesia, one of the operating room nurses will monitor your vital signs and make your *intraoperative stay* (time in surgery) as comfortable as possible. Either your surgeon, or the nurse, will start an I.V. In addition to the standard noninvasive monitors, you may receive supplemental oxygen through a soft plastic tube resting at the tip of your nose.

Using a small needle, your surgeon will slowly inject the local anesthetic into the surgical site. No matter how carefully the local anesthetic medication is injected, it may be somewhat painful for you. Your surgeon may direct the nurse to administer small doses of sedative medications through your I.V. at this time to help make you more comfortable. However, you will not be completely asleep and may recall much of the intraoperative course. This anesthetic technique is called *local anesthesia with conscious sedation.*

After your surgery, the length of recovery time necessary before you are discharged home will depend upon how much sedation you required and whether or not you experience postoperative nausea and unsteadiness. Generally, you can be discharged into the company of a responsible adult who has received instructions about your postoperative care shortly after termination of the procedure. However, be aware that even though you only had a local anesthetic, you may still require assistance at home for a short time until you are fully recovered from the anesthetic medications.

Surgery Under Local Anesthesia
With an Anesthesiologist Present

In this case, the main anesthetic is still the local anesthetic injected by the surgeon directly into the operative site. As with the previously discussed local anesthesia technique, it is limited in application to relatively simple surgical procedures in a suitable anatomic location.

The difference is that instead of a nurse monitoring you, an anesthesiologist is present during the entire surgical procedure to monitor you and administer intravenous sedatives to keep you comfortable. An anesthesiologist's expertise is needed either because a relatively large amount of sedation is necessary to keep you comfortable, or because your overall medical condition warrants constant vigilance by the anesthesiologist in order to ensure your safety.

This anesthetic technique is also called *local anesthesia with I.V. conscious sedation.* The intravenous sedative medications are meant to supplement the local numbing medications.

The intravenous sedative medications most commonly used for these type of procedures include representatives from several classes or categories of drugs. One category of drug often given is a *narcotic.* Examples of a narcotic include *Fentanyl, Demerol,* or *morphine.* These are analgesic (pain relieving) medications which are given to both supplement the action of the local anesthetic and provide a sense of well-being and relaxation during the surgery. They are painlessly administered through the I.V. in small, incremental doses throughout the duration of your surgical procedure. The anesthesiologist will carefully adjust the amount and timing of administration so that you are continuously relaxed and comfortable.

Some patients experience mild nausea associated with one or more of the narcotic drugs. If this is a problem for you, the anesthesiologist can give another drug (*anti-emetic*) intravenously to combat nausea.

Another class of drugs often used for conscious sedation are the benzodiazepenes. Drugs in this category include *Valium*, *Versed*, *Halcion*, and *Ativan*. Each drug in this class has the overall effect of reducing anxiety, and causing mild sedation and amnesia for the time period the drugs are in effect. Each drug also has its own specific, main effect. Halcion is primarily used to combat insomnia (a *sleeping pill*); Valium is prescribed to alleviate anxiety (a *tranquilizer*); and Versed is used in the operating room because it produces a rapid mild sedation and a sense of relaxation.

Versed wears off very quickly, within an hour or two, and does not produce nausea. When it is given in combination with the narcotic drugs, the pattern of breathing is altered so that the patient breathes less deeply and at a slower rate. In this instance, supplemental oxygen is usually administered through a soft plastic tube placed at the patient's nose or mouth. The anesthesiologist will constantly monitor the patient's oxygen level, adequacy of respirations, heart rate, and rhythm to ensure the patient's safety and comfort.

Occasionally, the anesthesiologist will administer very small doses of a drug called *propofol* through the patient's intravenous line. Propofol causes greater sedation than Versed but also wears off very quickly. It is only administered by an anesthesiologist because it may alter respirations to the point that the anesthesiologist must assist the patient's breathing with a mask.

When the surgical procedure is over, if you have received local anesthesia or local anesthesia with conscious sedation, you must still spend a certain amount of time in the recovery room. Staff will continue to monitor you until the peak effect of the sedating drugs has diminished, you are not nauseated, the pain from the surgery is minimal, and there is no excessive bleeding from the surgical site. This usually requires a minimum stay of one hour after the completion of surgery, but on occasion it can take longer.

When the staff determines you are stable enough to go home, you must be discharged into the hands of a responsible adult. This person must have received and understood your post operative instructions, be able to drive you home or accompany you in a cab, and stay with you for the next 12 to 24 hours. If you do not have a responsible adult to look after you, the staff will require you to stay overnight in their facility or hospital. By the next day, the effects of the I.V. anesthetics will have disappeared completely.

Under no circumstances should you plan on driving a car on the same day of your surgery if you receive the types of drugs discussed above.

General Anesthesia

The very idea of general anesthesia, which by definition implies a complete loss of consciousness and loss of ability to protect one's airway from aspiration, is terrifying for many people. However, under certain circumstances it is the best (or possibly the only) option for anesthesia. General anesthesia is required when the anesthetic technique must produce a state of sleep so deep (for example, a coma) that the patient is not affected by the pain of the operation.

Consider how quickly you would awaken if someone were to attack you with a knife while you were sleeping normally. During your operation, the surgeon must be able to perform your surgical procedure without you awakening. This means the general anesthetic state is not like your usual night-time sleep state. It is a much deeper state of sleep, carefully induced by the agents the anesthesiologist administers. It is important to remember that the combination of modern monitoring techniques and safe, effective anesthetic agents (drugs), used by the highly trained anesthetists make general anesthesia a much safer and more pleasant experience than ever before.

The amount of pain produced during surgery varies by procedure. Since not all surgeries cause the same amount of pain, not all surgeries require the same depth of anesthesia-induced sleep. The depth of anesthesia is determined by a number of factors including the patient's vital signs and the type of surgical stimulation occurring at various times in the operation. The anesthesiologist has the expertise necessary to determine the exact type and amount of anesthesia each patient requires for every phase of the surgical procedure.

Some of the anesthetic agents will be carefully administered through the patient's intravenous line, either as small, repeated doses or as a continuous, steady infusion. Other anesthetic agents are inhaled as gases. These gases are inhaled continuously during the surgery. They are administered either through a breathing tube the anesthesiologist inserts into the patient's airway after the patient is asleep or through a soft mask placed over the patient's face.

All agents given to induce a state of general anesthesia alter the normal pattern of breathing. Depending upon the specific surgical requirements and the agents used, the patient will either breathe spontaneously (on his or her own) but more rapidly and with shallow breaths, or will not breathe spontaneously at all.

Some type of *respiratory support* (breathing assistance via a mask or ventilator) is always required to ensure the patient receives an adequate amount of oxygen and eliminates an adequate amount of carbon dioxide.

Throughout the surgery, the anesthesiologist will constantly monitor the levels of oxygen and carbon dioxide in your blood. This is usually done with a non-invasive monitoring technique such as the pulse oximeter discussed earlier in this chapter.

Some of the anesthetic agents as well as some types of surgical procedures will cause changes in the patient's heart rhythm or rate. A continuous EKG or electrocardiogram (heart monitor) is always used to pick up any changes in the heart's rate or rhythm. Most of these changes are very benign and easily treated with medications the anesthesiologist administers through the IV.

Depending upon which anesthetic agents are used, general anesthesia may also cause alterations in the patient's blood pressure. These changes are usually not life-threatening and sometimes do not require any treatment. For those patients already suffering from hypertension (chronic high blood pressure), wider fluctuations in blood pressure are often seen and may continue into the immediate postoperative recovery period. In this case, the anesthesiologist can control the patient's blood pressure with medications injected through the I.V. If the patient's blood pressure is extremely high or low before surgery, the anesthesiologist may advise postponing the operation until a more acceptable blood pressure is achieved with oral medications. This prevents complications from arising during or after surgery.

What are the general *anesthetic agents* (medications) used? By definition, anesthesia includes *analgesia* (pain relief); *amnesia* (loss of memory for the event); and *sedation* (relaxation or sleep). The earlier anesthetic agents used, for example ether, adequately provided all three of these factors in a single agent but with many undesirable side effects. Problems included the potential for the ether to explode; a very long duration of action (long-lasting effect); difficulty in making fine adjustments to anesthetic depth; intense nausea and vomiting during the recovery period; and an undesirable drop in blood pressure.

In fact, if someone relates an old story about a patient in the distant past who "was allergic to general anesthesia and either had great difficulty waking up or never woke up," it is probably not that the unfortunate patient was truly allergic to the anesthetic, but rather that they suffered from an unintentional overdose of these difficult to manage agents. Things have improved radically — not just in the past twenty years — but even more so in the last five to 10 years.

Ideally, an agent would have absolutely no side effects, be easy to administer, and have a short duration of action. Although no such ideal agent yet exists, we have several that approach the ideal. The agents used today are much safer and have very few side effects.

To achieve the most desirable anesthetic effect, the anesthesiologist will usually use several agents in combination. This is because each agent contributes a unique action to the overall anesthetic state. First, a sedating agent, such as *sodium pentothal* or propofol, is administered through the patient's I.V. to gently begin inducing the deep sleep of general anesthesia.

These two drugs cause unconsciousness very quickly when given intravenously; however, their duration of effect is short. Sodium pentothal is not used in a repeated fashion and propofol is only sometimes used in a continuous low dose infusion to help maintain anesthesia. These two drugs are also limited by the fact that they do not provide any pain relief or amnesia. Therefore, other agents are needed to maintain anesthesia and provide amnesia and pain relief.

To achieve these additional desired effects, incremental doses of a narcotic (for example, Fentanyl or Demerol) and *anesthetic gases* (e.g. *Halothane, Forane,* or newer agents combined with nitrous oxide) mixed with a high concentration of oxygen are administered. In addition, a muscle relaxant is frequently given throughout the procedure to relax tissues and provide optimal operating conditions (for example, during abdominal surgery). Sometimes local anesthetics are also injected into the surgical site by the surgeon which may necessitate adjustments to the general anesthetic requirement.

Keeping all this in mind, one can see that today it would be very difficult to receive an overdose of any agent during general anesthesia because the anesthesiologist continually monitors your vital signs and each drug is given in very small, carefully calculated amounts throughout the surgery.

The general anesthetic agents used today still have some undesirable side effects. A certain percentage of patients will suffer nausea postoperatively. Among those particularly at risk for this are patients who have a history of motion sickness; a history of postoperative nausea with prior surgeries; a history of middle ear surgery; or those undergoing laparoscopic surgery.

This nausea can usually be easily dealt with by giving small amounts of safe anti-emetics via the intravenous line. To prevent nausea in the recovery period, the anesthesiologist will often give anti-emetics *prophylactically* during surgery to those patients who are at the highest risk of having postoperative nausea.

Another undesirable effect of anesthesia seen in the recovery room is shivering. No one knows why patients shiver after anesthesia, although it is thought to be due to a temporary alteration in the brain's ability to regulate the body's temperature. Shivering can occur even if the patient's temperature is close to normal after surgery.

Despite the cool temperature in the operating room, the anesthesiologist makes every attempt to keep you warm during the operation. Techniques include keeping all body parts not in the surgical area covered with a warming blanket, warming the gases you breathe, and warming the intravenous fluids flowing through the I.V. line.

In the recovery room, you can be kept warm with warming blankets and warming lights. The anesthesiologist may also prescribe a small dose of Demerol to be given via I.V. This often eliminates shivering completely, although why Demerol has this effect is still unknown.

Contrary to popular belief, there are generally no long-lasting side effects from general anesthesia. Patients who are basically healthy usually recover rapidly. However, it is important to remember that the patient must recover from both the anesthetic and the surgery itself.

If the surgery was very complex or of long duration, the recovery period will be prolonged and the patient should expect to feel drowsy and weak for a few days. For most outpatient procedures, the patient can expect to feel drowsy for several hours and perhaps even for part of the following day.

Patients who are very old, very frail, or have serious medical problems (for example, a history of stroke or heart attack) have an additional risk of longer lasting changes in mental status (confusion).

The American Society of Anesthesiologists has developed a standardized classification system to determine a patient's overall risk of complications from anesthesia and surgery. This is based upon the patient's overall health before surgery. The risk categories range from *ASA 1*: very low-risk such as a patient with either no disease or very minimal underlying disease (for example, a healthy patient who needs gall bladder surgery) to *ASA 5*: extremely high-risk such as a patient who is already comatose and has a life-threatening condition (for example, an unconscious patient suffering from multiple, severe gunshot wounds).

Those patients who have a serious medical problem (aside from the surgical problem) but have them under reasonable control with medication, are in a moderate risk category (for example, a patient with a history of chronic hypertension, angina, stroke, heart attack, diabetes, or emphysema requiring gall bladder surgery). This type of patient has a higher risk of sustaining another heart attack, stroke, or respiratory problem in the operative or immediate postoperative period.

Regional Anesthesia

In some instances, other anesthesia techniques are offered to the patient. These techniques can only be used for certain types of surgeries and usually only if the surgery is expected to last a short or moderately short amount of time. This type of anesthesia is called *regional* anesthesia and includes *spinal anesthetic*, *epidural anesthetic*, and specific nerve blocks such as a *brachial plexus block* for carpal tunnel syndrome.

A spinal or epidural anesthetic can be used for lower extremity and some lower abdominal surgeries (e.g., Cesarean section delivery). Epidural anesthesia is often used during childbirth to alleviate the pain of uterine contractions and to provide comfort during a vaginal delivery. An epidural can also be used to treat some types of postoperative surgical pain.

Even when you are to receive a regional anesthetic, the anesthesiologist will still place an intravenous line preoperatively. This ensures that intravenous fluids, mild sedatives, and any necessary emergency drugs can be easily administered. All the usual monitors will be placed to watch blood pressure, heart rate, oxygen level, and other indicators. Then you will be assisted to sit upright or to lie on your side in a curled up position.

Your lower back will be washed with an antiseptic solution and the anesthesiologist will use a very tiny needle to inject a numbing medicine into the skin directly over the site selected for injecting the main anesthetic. Once the skin is numb, another small needle will be placed in the lower back between the spinal bones. The anesthesiologist is highly skilled at placing this needle. He or she will insert it slowly and with great care, guided entirely by the feel of the needle tip as it advances through soft tissue and ligaments. It is usually not a painful procedure, but may take longer if the patient is elderly and has calcified spinal ligaments or has scar tissue from previous back surgery, because both conditions sometimes make it more difficult for the anesthesiologist to feel the needle as it advances.

A larger dose of local anesthetic will then be injected through this needle either into the space just outside the covering of the spinal cord (epidural) or injected into the center of the spinal cord and mixed with the spinal fluid (spinal anesthetic).

With an epidural, a very small, soft plastic tube is left in the spinal area so that additional, repeated injections of anesthetic can be administered. You will not have any discomfort from this epidural catheter. In the case of a spinal, the needle is removed. In either case, you will be assisted to lie back on the operating table and within a few minutes your legs and, if necessary, lower abdomen will become numb.

The anesthesiologist remains with you for the duration of the surgery to insure that you are always safe and comfortable. Often, supplemental anesthetic agents will be administered intravenously during the surgery to make the surgical experience easier for you.

Recovery from this type of regional anesthetic may take one to three hours or so, depending upon the type of local anesthetic agent used. Since this type of anesthetic may temporarily alter the blood pressure, you can expect to stay in the recovery room until the numbing effects of the anesthesia have worn off.

Many people fear there is a high risk of being paralyzed for life after a spinal anesthetic. In large-scale studies done over many years, the risk of spinal or neurological complications after a spinal anesthetic has been shown to be less than .04 percent, or less than 4 in 10,000 patients. In the overwhelming majority of patients who showed any kind of neurologic change, it was determined that there was actually some sort of pre-existing neurologic problem which became aggravated postoperatively.

A much more common postoperative complaint following a spinal anesthetic is a severe headache. This is often called a *spinal headache* and can be expected in about 10 out of 100 patients. The incidence is especially high in pregnant women and progressively less common in patients over 70 years of age. The risk of a spinal headache is not different if the patient lies flat on their back following surgery or gets up and moves about soon after surgery. If the headache is going to occur, it will present on the first or second day following surgery and spontaneously subside after four or five days.

The incidence of spinal headaches has decreased significantly with the now common use of very small gauge (very tiny and fine) spinal needles. Also, should you suffer a spinal headache, the anesthesiologist can offer a greater than 90 percent cure for the headache with a technique called an *epidural blood patch*. This simple procedure can be easily performed at your bedside after surgery.

Conclusion

Remember, the ultimate decision about what type of anesthetic is best for you is based on many factors, including your overall health, the type of surgery planned, and the length of the surgical procedure. Do not be afraid to state your preference or to ask questions about the various anesthetic options. However, keep an open mind as you discuss your options with your surgeon and anesthesiologist. Your anesthesiologist has the experience and expertise to develop an individualized anesthesia plan especially for you. This will ensure that your surgery is accomplished in the safest, most comfortable way possible.

CHAPTER NINE

Those First Few Moments:
The Operating Room Experience

Scenario

You are scheduled for surgery today. Your bedside alarm clock goes off and you quickly reach over and turn it off. Setting the alarm was unnecessary this morning because you've been awake for hours, mentally reviewing all the details you must attend to before undergoing your operation.

Your mother is coming to help take care of the kids; you've got a week's supply of groceries in the cupboards; and your sick leave at work has been approved. You know what the insurance company is going to pay for, and the clerk in the hospital admitting department has assured you that your paperwork is all in order.

Everything and everyone is taken care of, and now it's time to focus on yourself. What should you be doing this morning? How can you prepare for your hospital or surgical center stay?

Most people like to shower, shave, and wash their hair so they start the day feeling fresh. Keep your hairstyle simple and neat. You may not feel like washing your hair again for several days (or may not have the opportunity), so avoid using lots of hair pins, hair spray, or gel.

On the day of surgery, women should keep the use of cosmetics to a bare minimum. Even if you are someone who normally refuses to leave the house without full makeup, please limit yourself to a very light touch of lipstick. Also remove any nail polish you may be wearing. The physicians and nurses can monitor your circulation by checking the amount of pinkness in your nailbeds and skin. They prefer to evaluate you without artificial blush, shadows, and nail polish in the way. Remember, hospital staff members are very accustomed to seeing people at less than their best.

Wear simple, comfortable clothes and shoes. A warm-up or jogging suit is usually a good choice, as are tennis shoes or flats. Avoid clothes that bind, are difficult to get into, or that wrinkle easily. After your surgery, you will not feel like fastening a long row of buttons or walking in shoes with high heels. Your clothes will probably be folded and stored in a big plastic sack or container of some sort until they're returned to you after the surgery (if you are being discharged home), or sent to your hospital room (if you are transferred to a nursing unit for further recovery).

If you must stay overnight in the hospital, a good rule of thumb is to bring only the basic necessities. Items to consider packing include:

- Toothbrush
- Toothpaste
- Denture case and fixative
- Contact lens case and solution
- Reading glasses
- Hair comb/brush
- Deodorant
- Slippers (Soft slippers with rubber soles are best.)
- Bathrobe (A kimono-style wrap robe that ties in front is best. Try to avoid bathrobes that must be stepped into. Also try to bring a robe that has large, loose sleeves instead of tight cuffs at the wrists or elbows.)
- Nightclothes (see following note)

Bringing your own nightgown or pajamas to wear during your hospital recovery may be an option, but please consider the following points. First, depending upon your operation, you may have tubes, drains, and bandages in place that make wearing regular bed clothes impossible. Perhaps you will be connected to a heart monitor or have temporary heart pacemaker wires in your upper abdomen. Sometimes there is wound drainage that will leak and stain your nightclothes, or you may perspire heavily and need frequent changes of damp nightclothes. In any of these situations, a hospital gown is best.

If you decide to bring your own bed clothes and you're a woman, your nightgowns must be sleeveless (or have very short sleeves) and should be knee length. One reason this is necessary is because the nurse must be able to apply the blood pressure cuff directly to your upper arm in order to accurately monitor your blood pressure. Also, if you have a simple intravenous line or need blood drawn, your arms must be uncovered so the veins can be accessed.

The nurse will also have to look at your surgical wound, bandages, and stitches several times throughout the day. If you have a chest or abdominal wound, and are wearing a long gown, it will make checking your bandages and wound much more difficult. Pulling a long gown up above your abdomen may actually result in exposing more of you than if you were wearing a hospital gown that can simply be folded back.

Men also should consider if they really need to bring their own pajamas because often they are not the best choice for sleepwear. It is much easier to manage in a hospital gown or "Johnny" gown, especially if the man has had urinary or prostate surgery that requires a tube be inserted into his bladder to drain urine (*urinary catheter*). It's very difficult to handle a catheter and the attached urine collection bag if it has to be run down inside a pajama leg. It's much simpler for the patient to navigate if the bag is strapped onto their bare leg and the collection bag pinned to the hem of a gown. In any case, should the Johnny gown be unsatisfactory, most hospitals have pajamas available for patient use.

Hospital staff understand it's important for you to feel that you look presentable. But keep in mind that you're in a hospital and no one expects you to feel perky or look gorgeous. Everyone understands how unexpectedly out of sorts people can feel after surgery.

Be careful: you don't want your choice of bedclothing to become a disincentive or obstacle for the staff to care for you. This is exactly what you want to avoid. Make it as easy as possible for both you and your caregivers to work around your bedclothes.

Every attempt is made to take good care of your personal belongings, but there are many opportunities for things to get misplaced. Avoid bringing anything expensive or irreplaceable. Leave all your jewelry at home. The one exception you can make is to wear your wedding band or some other small sacred item that you feel you cannot part with.

The staff will make every effort to allow you to keep your wedding band or religious medal. Ask to have your ring taped in place on your finger. If you want to wear a religious medal, discuss this with the staff and ask how they recommend you accomplish this. Usually, any type of necklace or neck chain is removed prior to surgery because the anesthesiologist must have unrestricted access to your neck and shoulders.

You have packed your bag, kissed everyone in the family good-bye, and been driven to the hospital or surgical center. You go to the preoperative area and sign-in with the receptionist. She snaps a plastic armband with your name and medical record number onto your wrist, asks your significant other to take a seat in the waiting room and walks you down a hall to either a small dressing room or behind a pulled curtain next to your bed. She hands you a neatly folded hospital gown, and a large plastic bag for your clothes.

"Please change into this hospital gown," she will tell you. "You may place your clothes into the plastic bag. Someone will be with you in a minute."

You quickly begin to undress. Two questions suddenly come to mind. Do you have to wear the hospital gown since you brought your own nightclothes? Should you remove your underwear?

The answer to both questions is "yes." All surgical patients are required to wear the knee-length, light cotton gown that ties in the back. These gowns are specifically designed to allow the staff easy access to the various areas of your body they must work on, and yet maintain as much privacy as possible for you.

The exact spot for your incision may be small, but the nurses will scrub a very wide area all around the surgical site with special soap. This large, well scrubbed area reduces the chance of infection by removing as many bacteria as possible from the surgical area. This soap is often brownish and would stain your clothes if you wore them, so remove all of your underwear, including a bra or any shorts, briefs, or panties. Anything other than the hospital gown is almost never allowed on the patient during surgery.

Once you have changed into your hospital gown, a staff member will return, state your name, introduce themselves to you, and double-check that your arm name band, your hospital card, and your record match. Then they will obtain your height and weight. This information is necessary because it helps the anesthesiologist calculate the dosages of drugs to give you during your operation.

After you have been weighed, they will ask you to use a small step stool to climb up onto a narrow bed which is called a stretcher or gurney. These beds have thin, narrow mattresses, are on wheels, and have metal side rails. This makes them easy to move. You will be wheeled into the operating room on this bed or gurney.

Make yourself comfortable, because you will not be going to the operating room for several more minutes. If you are cold, ask for an extra blanket. If you want the bed adjusted, ask to have the head raised. The only thing you must not do is ask for a drink of water. Your stomach must be entirely empty when you go to the operating room.

After listing your belongings and making certain your wallet and other valuables are either given to a family member or friend or safely put away, the staff may ask you if you have brought any paperwork from the surgeon. Some physicians send the documents with the patient, while others fax the papers or send them ahead of time. Do not be concerned if you don't have any paperwork with you. But if you do have papers, now is the time to hand them over to the staff.

There will be a last-minute verification of your admission or pre-registration information, your insurance coverage, and your laboratory tests. The staff must be certain that any tests or X-rays you had done are noted in the record and that the results are also recorded. Sometimes you may need a few additional tests and a laboratory technician will come to collect more blood or urine.

Unless you pre-signed your papers, the staff will need to complete the final paperwork. They will ask you about your surgical procedure and your understanding of what the operation is all about. It's important for them to know that you are well informed before you sign the document giving your permission for the operation to take place.

Your temperature, pulse, and blood pressure will be taken, and then you will be asked if you wear glasses, contact lenses, a hearing aid, dentures, or artificial arms or legs. In almost all cases, these items will have to be removed before you are moved to the operating room.

You will be asked about your medical history – again. You have already answered most of the questions during your visits to the surgeon and anesthesiologists as well as during your preoperative assessment examination. However, you will be asked one more time as a safety check.

Many times the staff will read through a list of medical problems such as lung problems, seizures, heart disease, hypertension, pacemakers, bleeding disorders, cancer, hepatitis, liver disease, diabetes, past surgeries, back or neck pain, or gynecological problems. They read this list in hopes that it will remind you of any problems you have, but you may have forgotten to mention. If you suffer from any of the problems they read to you, be certain to tell them.

They will also ask you if you are using tobacco, alcohol, or recreational street (illicit) drugs. Be honest because these things can cause unexpected reactions in your body while you are under anesthesia. These are health care professionals who want to provide you with safe care during your operation. They are not making moral judgments on your behavior.

They will note if you have any kind of vision or hearing impairment. They want to be certain that if they remove your hearing aid you can still understand what is happening in surgery and will be able to have your questions answered. They will also determine if you need an interpreter if your primary language is not English.

They will observe how you move onto the gurney. This helps them plan your transfer from the operating room table back onto the gurney and then later into a hospital bed if necessary. If you have any special needs, chronic problems, or difficulty moving it is a good idea to tell the staff about it now. It helps them plan how they can best support you while you are with them in the hospital.

Next you will be asked again to tell them what medications you are currently using. They want to know the name of the drug, why you take it, how much you take, and how often. They will also want to know when you took your last dose. It's very helpful if you write this information down beforehand or use our medication list form at the end of Chapter 12. Then you can just hand your list to the staff member.

They will also read a fairly comprehensive list of medications and ask you if you have ever had any allergies or sensitivities to these medications. Remember, they want to know about any skin rashes, wheezing, nausea, facial swelling, or other problems associated with medications you have taken.

Drugs on their list often include *antibiotics* such as *penicillin*, *gentamicin*, *sulfas*, and pain medications such as *morphine*, *codeine*, *Demerol*, *Dilaudid*, *Darvon*, or *Talwin*. They may ask about aspirin, Motrin, Nuprin, and other anti-inflammatories. Numbing medicines like novocain and xylocaine, tranquilizers like *Valium*, and other *sedatives* or *barbiturates* may also be included. In addition, they may ask you about allergies to *diagnostic dyes* used in X-rays, adhesive tape, and allergies to foods, such as shellfish, eggs, peanuts, or strawberries.

The staff will quietly assess how nervous you are about your operation, and determine if you have anyone at home who will be supportive postoperatively. During this conversation they will again evaluate if you understand why you are having surgery and what your recovery will be like.

Once their operating room checklists are completed, they will verify one more time the site of your surgery. It's extremely important that you take a minute and think clearly to make certain you tell them exactly where your operation is to take place. Be very, very specific. For example, you should say, "I'm having surgery on my left knee, right here by the kneecap," rather than, "I'm having knee surgery." Many surgical staff are now asking the patient to mark the surgical site on their skin with a marker if the procedure involves the right or left side of the body.

Once all these questions have been answered (and if time allows), the staff will frequently ask if you would like the family member or friend who escorted you to the hospital or surgical center to sit at your bedside. You are now in the final stages of your surgical preparation. However, there may be another waiting period until the anesthesiologist or surgeon is ready for you. You may find it comforting to have a loved one spend this time with you.

A few minutes before you are wheeled into the operating room, the anesthesiologist who will assist with your operation may come into your room to say hello. (Note: Other times you will be introduced in the operating room.) At this time, if the anesthesiologist has not done an assessment prior to this day of surgery, last-minute questions about your past medical history and your previous experience with anesthesia will be gone over. He will also start an intravenous line so fluids and medications can be administered quickly and easily.

An intravenous line (I.V.) consists of a clear, soft plastic bag filled with fluid and a long length of plastic tubing attached to the bottom of the bag. A small needle will be inserted directly into the center of one of your veins, and the tubing will be attached to the outside end of the needle.

You may experience a brief moment of discomfort as the needle pierces your skin, but once that's accomplished you should not feel pain. The needle and tubing will be securely taped in place. You will be able to move your arm or hand, but it's important that you avoid disturbing your I.V., because if the needle becomes dislodged from the center of the vein it will have to be reinserted.

The operating room nurse who will assist the surgeon with your operation may also come to your bedside for a few minutes. This person will then review your medical record, and make a last minute check on when you last ate or drank. You were probably told not to eat or drink anything after a specific time (for example, midnight) the evening before your surgery. This is extremely important because the anesthesia must be given to you on an empty stomach to avoid any problems with vomiting. If you have had *anything* to eat or drink – even a few sips of water or a pill – tell the nurse what you had and the approximate time. The nurse will discuss this with the anesthesiologist, and they will decide if it is safe to proceed with your procedure as planned, or if it is best to delay your surgery for a few hours.

The operating room nurse will give you a paper shower cap to pull over your hair and will double-check to make certain your dentures, glasses, and other personal items have been properly stored. Then the nurse and either an assistant or the anesthesiologist will raise the side rails on your gurney, release the brakes, and begin to transport you to the operating room.

If the patient is a child, this final check by the operating room nurse may be different. Parents are frequently allowed to stay with their child from the moment they come into the hospital until the time their pre-operative medication has made them very sleepy. Only when the child is relaxed will the operating room nurse or physician carry the child into the operating room. This procedure probably won't relieve the parents' anxiety, but it's the least traumatic for the child.

You lie on your gurney and gaze up at the passing ceiling tiles as you are quickly wheeled along the corridor. "This is it," you think to yourself. Here is what you can expect.

Large doors swing open, and suddenly you are in a cool, brightly lit room. There may be soft music playing but it still seems very busy and crowded. You notice a narrow table in the middle of the room with large lights over it and several more tables along the edges of the room.

The tables along the sides of the room are draped with large tablecloths, and you may be able to see row after row of gleaming stainless steel instruments as the staff efficiently opens up several wrapped packages and neatly lines the contents up on the tables. These instruments and tabletops are sterile. They have been subjected to a process that has killed all of the germs (*contaminants*) on the instruments.

Everyone seems to be dressed identically in simple cotton uniforms (*scrubs*) and everyone is wearing a hat, perhaps just like the one you were asked to wear. Everyone's nose and mouth is covered by a face mask. All these special clothes help to prevent germs from entering the operating room.

Seeing this high level of activity and the masked strangers can be a very frightening experience. Remember, the operating room nurse and other members of the team are there to help you. If you could use a little reassurance, let them know.

Your surgeon may or may not be in the room at this point. In fact, you may have passed him in the hallway of the operating room where he was standing at a sink scrubbing his arms and hands. This wash is called a surgical scrub. A special antiseptic soap is lathered over the arms and hands and then scrubbed with a small brush for about ten minutes. It is a standard procedure done to clean the operating room staff's hands and forearms of bacteria, dirt, dead skin cells, and other germs.

As staff complete their scrub they do not use a regular towel to dry their arms and hands. Instead, they enter the operating room and are carefully provided with a sterile towel. You may notice a few people standing in a corner of your room drying their hands. After their hands are dry, they are assisted into a second gown that covers their scrub uniform. This is a long-sleeved cotton gown with tight-fitting, knit cuffs. Sterile gloves are pulled on over their hands and over the cuffs of the gown. This way, they are completely covered in sterile clothes when they do your operation.

The staff dress in sterile clothes to protect you. Your skin is a natural barrier that keeps harmful bacteria out of your body. When skin is cut or punctured during an operation, the natural barrier is opened, and bacteria may have the opportunity to enter your body and cause an infection. Wearing sterile clothes and using sterile instruments limits the number of bacteria around and in your open wound. This decreases the chance of any harmful bacteria entering your body.

The anesthesiologist and one of the operating room nurses (known as the circulating nurse) will position your gurney alongside the narrow table in the middle of the room. This is the operating table. They will ask you to assist them in transferring you over onto this table. Move carefully; there's no need to rush.

The operating table is very hard and will feel cool. Once there, you may be given pillows to make your head and knees more comfortable. Staff will also strap a loosely-fitting Velcro belt around your waist to remind you to stay in the center of the table.

The anesthesiologist will take a blood-pressure reading and probably will leave the cuff loosely wrapped around your upper arm. He will explain what you and he will be doing over the next few minutes. This may include asking you to hold a rubber or plastic mask over your nose and mouth so that you can take a few deep breaths of oxygen. If your I.V. was not started in the preoperative area, it will be started now. A small clamp may be positioned onto a fingertip to monitor your oxygen level. It will not hurt.

While the anesthesiologist is talking to you, the nurses will be busy positioning you for your operation. They will position your arms along special boards attached to the operating table so you will be comfortable during surgery and also so that the flow of fluid running through your I.V. will not be obstructed. They will loosely strap your arms onto these boards so they won't move while you're asleep.

Depending upon your type of surgery, staff may add various parts to the operating table, or reposition your back, head, or legs. The anesthesiologist will untie your hospital gown at the neck so he can apply the heart monitor leads to your chest. Remember, none of this will hurt. Take a deep breath and try to relax.   The anesthesiologist will give you some medication either through an oxygen mask or your I.V. Whichever route he chooses, it will not cause any discomfort. You will fall asleep very quickly. If you are asked to count backward from 100 you probably won't reach 95 before you are blissfully asleep. Before you know it, you'll be waking up in the recovery room.

What happens to you from this point on? Once you are asleep, the anesthesiologist will insert a tube into your windpipe to keep your airway open and oxygen flowing into your lungs. The nurse will expose only your surgical site while keeping the rest of you covered. She will then thoroughly scrub a wide area with special antiseptic soap to cleanse your skin of any bacteria. She will begin with the incision site and then scrub in ever widening circles out to the sides of your body. This is done for several minutes to ensure that the vast majority of bacteria are removed. This helps prevent any wound infections as you recover, and also removes any skin oil that may interfere with the adhesion of bandages.

Once you have been positioned for surgery and your skin has been scrubbed, the surgeon will carefully position several sterile towels around the site of your incision. This is called *draping*. A cloth curtain will be placed between the surgical site and the anesthesiologist who will remain seated at your head, carefully monitoring your breathing, blood pressure, and pulse. The ceiling lights will be focused on the only part of you that is still exposed: your exact surgical site. Your operation is about to begin.

CHAPTER TEN

Post-Anesthesia Care: Waking Up

The operating room team (your nurses and physicians) will carefully transfer you from the operating room table onto a gurney after completion of your surgical procedure. This movement from one position to another may increase your heart rate and change the flow of blood through your blood vessels, resulting in an increase or decrease in your blood pressure and pulse rate. Because of this potential change in your vital signs, the physicians and nurses will closely monitor your blood pressure, pulse, and respirations during this time. They will also take care that your I.V. and any other tubes or catheters you may have in place are not disturbed.

The nurse anesthetist or anesthesiologist and one of the other staff members who helped with your surgery will transport you on the gurney to another area where you will be very closely watched. The extent of your surgery, and the amount of time it is anticipated will be required for your body's functions to return to normal, determines if the area you are transported to is the *Intensive Care Unit (ICU)* or the *Post Anesthesia Care Unit* (*PACU*, often referred to as the *recovery room*). Unless your surgical procedure was very complex, or your condition very unstable, you will go to the PACU.

The PACU is usually located adjacent to the operating room so the surgeons and anesthesiologists are not required to leave the surgical area, yet are close by in case unexpected changes in your condition require their assistance.

You may or may not remember being transported to the PACU. In fact, you may not remember any of your PACU experience, depending upon the type of anesthesia you are given. However, since we believe knowledge is critical to your well-being, we have chosen to give you detailed information about this aspect of your surgical care. Knowing about PACU activities will allow you to prepare questions for your anesthesiologist. Also, sharing this information with the family members or friends who will accompany you on the day of your surgery helps them understand what is happening to you during the time period between the actual operation and when they see you again.

Admission to the PACU

The PACU is a large, open room without interior walls. It is designed like this to allow the staff unobstructed observation and quick access to all patients. In most surgical facilities, the PACU is staffed primarily with registered nurses (RNs), perhaps licensed vocational nurses (LVNs), and certified nursing assistants (CNAs). To ensure your safety, one of these staff members will be at your bedside, or within a few steps of you, at all times.

These staff members are busy preparing for your arrival in PACU while you are still on the operating room table. If you had general anesthesia, the PACU time period is an extremely vulnerable time for you because you may still be unconscious or in a semi-conscious state and therefore unable to breathe effectively. They set up and ready any equipment or devices necessary to monitor and maintain your vital signs, I.V.s, or other tubes and catheters after surgery.

This high-tech equipment is kept in the PACU and, if you are awake, you will not only see many blinking lights, digital read-outs, buttons, and wires, but will also hear assorted beeps, buzzes, and chimes. These sights and sounds are all part of the cardiac monitors, oxygen delivery systems, pulse oximeters, sequential compression devices, and other pieces of machinery the staff use to monitor your condition. Please remember that none of these devices cause any pain or discomfort if used on you.

The OR team will push your stretcher or gurney into your assigned space, set the parking brakes, and tell the PACU nurse who will be caring for you about your surgical procedure, how well you tolerated the operation, and if any difficulties were encountered.

PACU Activities

As your PACU nurse receives the report about you and your surgical procedure from the OR team, the nurse or another PACU staff member will be simultaneously attaching the appropriate monitoring devices to you. Your blood pressure, pulse, respirations, and level of consciousness will be immediately assessed.

These same vital signs will be re-checked every five minutes for the first 15 or 20 minutes you are in the PACU. If you are stable, monitoring will decrease to every 15 minutes for an hour or so. Then you will be checked every 30 minutes until you are stable and ready for discharge from the PACU. In addition, your temperature will be taken and, if normal, will be checked hourly while you are in the PACU.

Your nurse will evaluate your level of consciousness by giving you simple commands, such as asking you to move your legs, wiggle your toes, or squeeze the nurse's hand. You will also be asked to determine if you have any pain and to describe the severity of it and where it is located.

As the nurse evaluates your vital signs and level of consciousness, the PACU nurse will also assess your I.V. lines to be certain they are patent and clear. The amount of I.V. fluids you are to receive will be mathematically calculated and any necessary adjustments to the flow rate will be made.

The nurse will examine any other tubes or catheters you may have in place (for example, a urinary catheter to drain urine from the bladder or a chest tube to drain air or fluid from the chest cavity) and will make certain they are not kinked or leaking so that they function properly. The nurse will check that the fluids draining from them are in appropriate amounts and of normal color and consistency. Our bodies are composed of a significant amount of fluid, so maintaining a close balance between fluids lost and fluids replaced is critical to your well-being.

The PACU nurse will also keep a close watch on your bandages. This may necessitate pulling back your blankets and lifting a corner of your hospital gown to get a direct look at the gauze and tape covering your incision.

Normally, the bandages will be clean or have just a small amount of blood-tinged fluid on them. If bright red fluid is seeping up through the bandage, this may be a sign of unusual bleeding. Often the nurse will use a marking pen to outline the bloody spot on your dressing and will re-check it frequently to see if the spot is enlarging. This indicates if the bleeding is continuing and, if so, the surgeon will be called to evaluate the situation.

Direct observation of a bloody bandage is not the only way the PACU nurse monitors you for unusual bleeding after surgery. Changes in your vital signs can also signal hidden blood loss. The PACU nurse will keep careful records of your vital signs in order to be aware of any trends in your statistics.

You will probably have a soft plastic tube placed next to your nose to deliver extra oxygen. Increased oxygenation and assistance with breathing will be provided until the anesthesia wears off and your body systems return to normal and full function.

Many patients arrive in the PACU from the operating room with an oral airway (plastic device that keeps the tongue from falling into the back of the throat and closing off the airway) in their mouth. If you are still asleep, you will probably have an oral airway in place.

As your anesthesia wears off, and you begin to wake up, the plastic airway will annoy you. Even though you are not fully awake, you will naturally push the oral airway out with your tongue. This is one of the first signs that you are awakening from the anesthesia and are capable of moving your tongue and keeping your airway open by yourself. If for some reason you are unable to remove the oral airway yourself, the nurse will remove it as you become more awake and alert so you don't gag.

Sometimes patients can have a reaction to the anesthesia or surgery that causes nausea and vomiting. The nurse will be at your side to assist you with an *emesis basin* and *suction catheter* if you become ill and vomit. Improvements in the anesthesia drugs and better anti-nausea medicines have helped control nausea and vomiting following surgery, but they still occasionally occur in the PACU.

The side rails to your stretcher will be raised and latched in the elevated position at all times while you are in PACU. This ensures that you don't accidentally roll out of bed as you begin to wake up. It also provides you with a handy tool to assist yourself with turning and repositioning if you want to change positions.

On certain occasions, a family member is allowed into the PACU to sit beside a stable patient. Generally, this is only permitted when the patient is a small child who awakens and is extremely anxious or uncomfortable and a parent or caregiver can alleviate some of the child's stress by holding and comforting him. The other situation when a visitor may come into the PACU to see a stable and awake patient is when the hospital has a policy stating patients undergoing certain types of surgery are to be kept overnight in the PACU. In this case, the family member or significant other is allowed into the PACU to see the patient.

Remember, these are exceptions to the "no visitors" policy of most PACU's. The average patient does not spend enough time in the PACU to necessitate visiting privileges, and in many cases is neither alert nor feeling well enough to want visitors.

Also, most PACU nurses have two major concerns about letting non-medical personnel into the PACU: invasion of privacy for the other patients and increased stress for the unprepared visitor.

The wide open design of the PACU makes it very difficult to protect the privacy of all the other patients when a visitor is allowed into the PACU. Although the patient to be visited may be stable, other patients may be unconscious, semi-conscious, or nauseated and uncomfortable.

Even if the patient to be visited is awake, most people are extremely pale immediately after surgery, attached to a variety of strange-looking monitoring devices, bandaged, or casted and have assorted I.V.s and tubing in place. Visitors, unprepared for the environment and the postop appearance of the patient, are unpleasantly surprised and become frightened because to them their loved one looks much worse than before surgery. If a distraught visitor suddenly feels "faint" it creates a situation that may temporarily pull the PACU staff's attention away from their PACU patients.

Common Patient Experiences in PACU

Patients who can remember PACU often have three common complaints about their experience: they feel cold, they have pain, and it is very noisy. Let's discuss each complaint so that if you experience the same things you will at least know why.

Cold

The operating room is kept at a much cooler temperature than the average room in your home. This is because the surgeons and staff must wear several layers of operating room clothing, including long-sleeved, sterile cover gowns. They also work under very bright and intense lights that generate a tremendous amount of heat. If the room is kept too warm, the required clothing and lights make it difficult for the surgeons to work.

You may also feel cold depending upon the type of surgical procedure you have. For example, sometimes when the patient is having an operation on a lower leg the surgeon must decrease the blood flow to that leg in order to perform the operation. A mechanical tourniquet is applied to temporarily decrease circulation to that limb. This may result in your leg feeling cooler for a few hours after surgery.

The PACU is prepared to quickly address your complaint of being cold. They have blankets that are kept in a heated cupboard or warming unit as well as large warming lights that can be used to raise your body's temperature. In some PACUs they have what is called a *"bair hugger,"* a controlled blanket that provides warm air over the patient. If you are cold, and one of these treatments is applied, you will feel warmer within minutes.

If your body temperature is normal, but you are shivering, the chills may be a side effect of your anesthesia. The PACU nurse will give you medication to counteract your symptoms and make you more comfortable. (*See Chapter 8 for more details about anesthesia.*)

Pain

Patients are generally still quite sedated when they begin to complain of pain. It's not unusual to have them wake up and complain of pain only to immediately fall asleep again. It's not always clear if they are truly experiencing pain or responding to the stress of surgery. Whenever you complain of pain, the PACU nurse will assess your condition by evaluating your vital signs, level of consciousness, and noting when you had your most recent pain medication and your response. Then the nurse will administer doses of pain medication as ordered by your surgeon. Usually this is a narcotic given in small doses through your IV line, so you will not feel the administration of the medication. Within a few minutes, your pain will be alleviated. You will doze and when you next awaken, you may feel more pain. Ask the nurse to reassess the situation and medicate you again as needed.

Noise

The equipment in the PACU that is used to monitor and maintain patients' stability can be very noisy. Each piece of machinery has an alarm and/or signal to help the staff evaluate your status. When each patient is attached to at least two of these beeping devices, and there are 10 or more patients in the open room of the PACU, the room can become very noisy. Patients who are awake in the PACU often comment that they are amazed the PACU staff can work in an environment with such a high noise level.

Discharge from PACU

When your vital signs are stable, you have not had any unexpected reactions to the surgery, you are awake and can respond appropriately to questions, your bandage has only minimal drainage, your urine output is sufficient, and your pain in under control, then you are ready for discharge from the PACU. If you had a regional anesthetic, you will also have to feel the beginning of sensation in the areas of your body adjacent to the operation.

Patients usually spend at least an hour in the PACU. Don't be alarmed if your stay is longer, and advise your family and friends that an extended stay in the PACU is not necessarily cause for alarm. Your time in the PACU can be influenced by a number of factors.

Some surgical facilities have a *step-down* or *phase II PACU*. In this area of the PACU unit, patients who have had same-day surgeries and are planning to go home are assisted to use the bathroom and helped to dress in their street clothes. They will then be asked to sit in a reclining chair and given a small amount of fluid to drink and perhaps a cracker to eat, just to be certain they don't suffer unexpected nausea and vomiting. Once the staff determines that vomiting and lightheadedness aren't a problem, and any pain is under control, the patient will be discharged into the care of the person who accompanied them. This phase II recovery may add another 30 minutes or more to your recovery time, depending upon how well you tolerate drinking fluids and sitting up.

Other reasons for a delay in your discharge from PACU include the following: your physician may order an X-ray or laboratory test and it takes several minutes for the technician and/or equipment to come to the PACU; you experience pain a few minutes before your scheduled transfer to the nursing unit, so the PACU nurse medicates you and now wants to monitor your response to the medication before transferring your care to the nurse on the unit; the nursing unit bed you are assigned to isn't ready; equipment needed to support your care at the nursing unit bedside hasn't been put in place; or it is change of shift time for the nursing unit staff, and the PACU nurse prefers to wait and give reports directly to the new shift. Any of these factors can delay your transfer out of the PACU, even when you are stable.

Once your PACU nurse believes you can be safely transferred to the nursing unit, she completes your records and calls the nurse who will be assigned to care for you on the unit. They will review your postoperative course, any questions will be answered, and the nurse on the unit will prepare your bed, set up your equipment and any medications or treatments your physician has ordered.

Staff from the PACU will transport you on your gurney to your assigned hospital room. There the staff will get you comfortably situated in your hospital bed, check your vital signs, and make certain your pain is under control. Your family will probably accompany you as you are moved from the PACU to the nursing unit or will be close behind the PACU team.

CHAPTER ELEVEN

What to Expect on the Nursing Unit

Scenario

Your physician has advised you that immediately after your operation it will be necessary for you to spend several days in the hospital. You have never been hospitalized before and wonder what to expect. We think the following information will help you prepare for this new experience.

After their surgical procedure, patients who are not discharged home will usually be admitted to a nursing unit, ward, or floor (all these terms are used interchangeably to describe patient care areas in the hospital). In some hospitals these units are dedicated to caring for patients with specific types of surgery, disease, or needs. For example, an orthopedic surgery unit primarily cares for patients who have had some type of orthopedic (bone) procedure, a respiratory ward is for patients with lung problems, and the labor and delivery unit is for women giving birth. Other hospitals combine the types of patients cared for in a designated area and these are called either medical or surgical units.

You will probably encounter several types of nursing staff on these units: registered nurses, licensed vocational nurses (also known as licensed practical nurses), and certified nursing assistants or hospital assistants.

A registered nurse has the most in-depth education. This person's basic academic preparation can range from a two-year

Associate of Arts degree, a three-year hospital school of nursing diploma, or a four-year Bachelor of Science degree. Some nurses have additional education leading to specialized certifications or advanced degrees such as a Master's degree. The RN has success-fully passed an extensive licensing test, and in many states must regularly complete several hours of continuing education in order to maintain an active license. All of this generally means the registered nurse has the most knowledge and understanding of pathophysiology and Nursing Science.

A registered nurse is a professional governed by the Nurse Practice Act and licensed to practice by the licensing board from the state in which this person works. Registered nurses are accountable to not only their supervisors, but also the hospital and the state board of registered nursing.

A licensed vocational nurse generally has one year of train-ing, and certified nursing assistants (also called *aides* or *orderlies*) have six or more weeks of training. All of these nursing staff per-sonnel also have clinical experience and on-the-job training in addition to their classroom preparation.

The ratio of nursing staff to patients is based upon the num-ber of patients on the unit, and also the acuity or amount of care each patient requires. A complicated mathematical formula is often used to calculate this ratio, which is adjusted for each shift.

The nurse manager of each unit is always a registered nurse. The remaining staff will consist of additional registered nurses, licensed vocational nurses, and certified nursing assistants.

Each registered nurse has ultimate responsibility for several patients. The RN must coordinate each patient's care and ensure that safe, therapeutic, high-quality nursing care is provided either directly by them or by those to whom they have delegated some aspects of care.

For instance, under the supervision of the RN, the LVNs and CNAs will often be assigned to take your vital signs, help you walk or sit at the side of the bed, assist you with bathing and personal care, assist you with postoperative exercises, complete specific procedures and treatments requested by your physician, and change your bed linens. This delegation of responsibilities often means you will see more of your LVN or CNA than you do your RN.

However, your RN is ultimately responsible for your care, and directly supervises the LVN and CNA assigned to you. The RN will evaluate your vital signs, activities, and other important parameters such as nutrition, fluid balances, lung sounds, and bowel function. This person is also responsible for monitoring your surgical incision site, bandages, intravenous lines, and any other drains or medical interventions and equipment. The RN prepares and administers all of your medications, including evaluating your level of pain and administration of pain medication as ordered by your physician. The RN evaluates your need for additional services from other hospital disciplines (for example, social services or dietary) and coordinates your care with these personnel.

Another of the RN's primary responsibilities is to develop a plan for your care that spans the period from your admission onto the unit until the time you are discharged. As such, the RN has a number of resources that can be used to assist you (for example, social workers, chaplaincy service, dietitians, physical therapists, occupational therapists, and respiratory therapists). The RN will work with your physician to be certain you have whatever is needed to help you achieve a rapid recovery.

It's very important that you make every effort to confide in your registered nurse any concerns you have regarding your care, condition, or recovery. Your RN is the primary communication link to your doctors and the point of coordination with other health care providers while you are in the hospital.

If for some reason you have difficulty communicating with one of your nurses, don't hesitate to seek out the nurse manager for the unit, who will be interested in knowing your concerns and will adjust the staff assignments to support your needs.

Nursing care must be provided on a 24-hour basis. Since one nurse cannot possibly work all 24 hours, the time is divided into shifts. Every time there is a shift change, there is a change of staff. The nurses' shifts overlap so that they can report to each other and ensure that your care is consistent. The off-going nurse makes certain the oncoming nurse is aware of your general status and any special circumstances or requirements you have.

The number of hours in a shift varies, with the most traditional being eight hour shifts: 7:00 a.m. to 3:00 p.m., 3:00 p.m. to 11:00 p.m. and 11:00 p.m. to 7:00 a.m.. Other possible variations are 10-hour shifts and 12-hour shifts. In any case, it is inevitable that you will have several different nurses responsible for your care. However, in most hospitals every attempt is made to provide some consistency for you by assigning the same nurses to care for you whenever they are on duty.

It is important for you to know that the "change of shift" overlap time is a time period when your nurses will be very busy completing paperwork and exchanging information about their patients' conditions with each other. They will not be as readily available to you for routine requests and care during their report time. This time generally lasts 30 to 45 minutes before the end of each shift. If you think you are going to need pain medication, help walking to the bathroom, or some other assistance during shift change, plan ahead and make your requests before change of shift begins.

Other hospital personnel available to assist you during your hospitalization include:

- *Physical therapist:* This professional develops an exercise therapy regime personalized for you. The physical therapist works with you during your hospital stay to help you strengthen muscles affected by your surgery or inactivity. Physical therapists also help you learn to move about with crutches or a walker and assist you with using a new artificial limb.

- *Occupational therapist:* If surgery has affected your ability to carry out activities of daily living (for example, dressing, eating, and personal care), this professional helps you develop or maintain adaptive skills to regain your physical independence. The occupational therapist will also make assistive devices or splints to help you regain function.

- *Respiratory therapist:* This professional will help you maintain adequate function in your lungs. The respiratory therapist may assist you with your coughing and deep breathing exercises, or help you use the respiratory machines that keep your lungs inflated and clear.

- *Clinical social worker:* This professional can provide you or your family with counseling as well as practical support to help you cope with the effects of your illness and hospitalization. A clinical social worker can give you information regarding support groups and services for your recovery at home.

- *Chaplainacy service:* These priests, ministers, rabbis, and specially trained lay people minister to various faiths and are usually available on an on-call basis. They contribute to the healing process by providing spiritual counseling, emotional support, prayer, and sacramental ministry to patients of all faiths. Many hospitals also have a chapel available in the hospital. Unless the hospital is affiliated with a particular denomination or faith, the chapel is non-denominational.

- *Pharmacy services:* The pharmacy department is staffed by licensed pharmacists, who are a valuable resource for information regarding any aspect of your medications. The pharmacist is the hospital's expert on medications. This person understands the actions, indications, contraindications, and adverse effects of all the drugs prescribed for you. If you are unclear about why you need certain medications, are uncertain about how to take them, or are already taking several medications and want to know how your new medications fit into your pre-surgery medication schedule, take advantage of this resource and ask to meet with a pharmacist prior to going home. (See Chapter 12 for additional information.)

- *Laboratory technician (phlebotomist):* This person is responsible for obtaining your blood samples when your physician orders tests on the contents of your blood. The "lab tech" will often come to your bedside to draw blood from a vein in your arm, placing it in small glass tubes to transport back to the clinical laboratory.

- *Radiology technician:* This person is responsible for taking and developing your X-rays. They will help position you for X-rays and will instruct you about movement and holding your breath so the pictures are clear and sharp.

As we mentioned earlier, your nurse will be carefully monitoring many aspects of your care to ensure a safe and quick recovery from your operation. The following areas are of particular importance and often of the greatest concern for patients.

Safety and Comfort

As soon as you arrive on the nursing unit from the PACU, your condition will be evaluated to be certain you are stable. First, your nurse will evaluate your respiratory status and make certain you are getting enough oxygen by observing the amount of pinkness in your nail beds and mucous membranes (skin lining the inside of your mouth and eyelids). She may ask you to cough and breathe deeply while listening to your lungs with a stethoscope. The extent of the respiratory evaluation will be determined by the type of surgery you had and the kind of anesthetic. The nurse determines if supplemental oxygen is needed. If it is, she will be certain it is ordered and administered to you through a plastic mask or soft nasal prongs.

Next the nurse will evaluate your cardiovascular system by taking your vital signs and evaluating the degree of moisture or dryness to your skin. Your pulse, blood pressure, and temperature will be taken and compared to the results of those obtained most recently in the PACU, and they will be checked to be certain everything is stable and as expected.

Next is a *neurological* check. She will determine your level of consciousness and ability to follow verbal commands. If you are still very sleepy, the side rails on your hospital bed will be locked in the upright position. She will then evaluate your surgical wound and bandages to be certain they are intact and there is no unusual drainage or problems. She will check any drainage tubes to be certain they are functioning and that fluids draining from them are the expected color, clarity, and amount.

She will check any other equipment you may have to support or monitor you. She carefully calibrates any monitoring equipment as appropriate and makes certain any connecting wires or lines are correctly attached. Every piece of equipment is thoroughly grounded so you do not have to worry that the wires and cords may present an electrical hazard.

You will be positioned in bed to avoid stress on your incision. This is often accomplished through the strategic placement of extra pillows or rolled blankets. Your nurse call bell will either be pinned to your gown or hooked to the side rail within easy reach. Your bedside table will be positioned so that you can easily reach your box of tissues, emesis basin, television control, and telephone.

If you are allowed to have ice chips, your nurse will make certain a cup of ice and spoon are positioned nearby. Take the ice chips slowly and infrequently. The action of your stomach and intestines may have been slowed down by the anesthetic drugs and therefore not functioning normally. If your gastrointestinal tract is sluggish, and fluids are not being absorbed as quickly as usual, taking too much fluid at once may cause nausea and vomiting. Pace yourself and take a small spoonful of ice chips every 15 or 20 minutes to help moisten your mouth and quench your thirst. If you begin to feel nauseated, stop taking ice chips and notify your nurse.

If you are not allowed to have ice chips, a mouth moistener on large swabs will be provided for you to wipe your lips and inside your mouth. Or your nurse may be able to offer you a mouthwash or other solution to swish for your dry mouth.

Pain Relief

We wish it wasn't true, but most patients will experience some discomfort after almost any surgical procedure. The amount of pain you experience will vary not only by the type of surgical procedure you undergo, but also by your individual perception of and ability to tolerate pain.

Your physician will prescribe pain medication to be given to you if you have pain. Keep in mind that regardless of the type of pain medication and its method of delivery, your discomfort is usually not totally relieved 100 percent of the time. However, pain medications can be quite effective when taken properly, so we would like to review some important points to help you maximize their effect.

The pain associated with uncomplicated major surgery is usually due to three factors: the surgical incision which irritates and cuts through nerve endings; the stretching and pulling of the tissues and muscles around the incision site; and the prolonged period of inactivity while you were on the hard operating room table.

You will be most aware of pain during movement, such as while sitting up, coughing, or repositioning yourself in bed. Providing support of the surgical site during movement is very helpful. This can be accomplished by holding a pillow snugly against your incision or placing one hand on each side of your incision to support the incisional area. Your nurse may refer to this as *splinting* your incision.

Pain medication is usually prescribed in one of two ways: every three or four hours as needed, or by a pain control intravenous machine.

Pain medication ordered "every three or four hours as needed" is exactly that: you will have to ask the nurse to prepare and administer your medication as you need it, but not more frequently than every three or four hours. This is usually the manner in which pain pills and injections (shots) are prescribed.

Many oral and injected pain medications will begin to exert an effect within about 20 minutes, reach their peak effectiveness within an hour, and will continue to provide relief (although with declining effectiveness) for about three to four hours. If one charts the effectiveness of pain medication, it usually looks like a bell-shaped curve.

It's important to keep this "peak and valley" effect of medication in mind as you take your pain medication. Taking your pain medication on a regular basis keeps a therapeutic level of medication in your blood, and you will probably find that this makes you most comfortable immediately after surgery.

If you are uncomfortable and need pain relief, don't hesitate to ask your nurse for pain medication. Pain medications, even strong narcotics, are seldom addictive when taken for the short amount of time they are needed after surgery. Also, it's not a sign of weakness if you find you need pain medication in order to walk, breathe deeply, and cough. It is very important that you are comfortable enough to change positions in bed frequently, carry out your postoperative exercises, and walk as soon after surgery as possible. All of this activity helps reduce the muscle discomfort, prevents lung complications, prevents pressure areas on your skin and aids your bowels and bladder to quickly return to normal function.

A *pain control machine* (PCA) is a type of specialized medical equipment which allows you, the patient, to self-medicate for pain. A pain relieving drug is mixed with an intravenous solution and then dispensed through the PCA machine into an intravenous line that has been inserted into one of your veins. You administer your own pain medication by simply pushing a button on the PCA machine. This releases a controlled and timed dose of pain medication into the I.V. line and allows you to maintain a steady blood level of pain medication. This avoids the peaks and valleys of relief often associated with taking pain medication on an every three-to-four-hour basis. The equipment is calibrated to ensure that no matter how frequently the machine's button is pushed, only a safe dose of pain medication will be administered. It is not possible to accidentally give yourself too much pain medication.

Nutrition

The need for proper nutrition in order to achieve rapid wound healing and prevent infection is well documented in the medical literature. A surgical procedure triggers a tremendous stress response in the body, resulting in a significant increase in metabolic demand. You simply need more energy to cope with the effects of surgery. In addition, a chemical chain of events may occur which negatively impacts your body's ability to function normally. At the very time you especially need additional nutrition your body may be unable to effectively metabolize foods into energy.

If you are in generally good health, you will be able to tolerate this insult to your body because you have a sufficient amount of body fuel reserved. This reserve enables you to withstand the metabolic insult and partial starvation caused by surgery. If you are older, debilitated, suffering from infections, have chronic problems, or are a child, you may not have the necessary nutritional reserve necessary to handle a complicated, extensive surgery that requires several days of hospitalization for recovery.

In these instances you will need additional dietary supplements, such as protein drinks or special intravenous fluids in addition to the regular diet and nutritional interventions.

Once you are able to tolerate ice chips without nausea, your physician will order what is called a progressive diet. This diet begins with clear liquids (for example, tea, broth, and jello) then progresses to a full liquid or soft diet (for example, hot cereal, milkshakes, poached eggs, and toast) and then onto a regular diet of your choice. If at any time you are unable to tolerate the foods in your diet, your nurse will make adjustments in the food selection. The nurse can solicit the advice of a dietitian or nutritionist to help you select foods that provide you with the nutrients necessary for healing.

Bowel Function

If you have had major abdominal surgery, your doctor or nurse probably told you that your bowels may react to the trauma of surgery by stopping their normal function. This temporary condition is called a *paralytic ilieus*. The symptoms include lack of bowel sounds (the normal rumbles and gurgles heard with a stethoscope as food moves through your intestines), lack of bowel movements and inability to pass *flatus* (gas). The degree of bowel function effected depends upon the location and extent of your surgery and how much manipulation or positioning of your bowels was required. Paralytic ilieus can also be due to a lack of mobility postoperatively, side effects of pain medications, and a reduction in fluid intake. A paralytic ilieus usually lasts only four to five days.

If you have a paralytic ilieus, you will not be given any foods to eat or liquids to drink. Instead, you will need to receive all of your nutrition and important *electrolytes* (potassium, calcium, magnesium, etc.) through your intravenous fluids. You will remain on intravenous feedings until your bowel function returns and you can once again process the foods and liquids you eat and drink. During this time, your blood will be checked regularly to be certain that your body's acids and bases are in balance and that you are receiving adequate vitamins and nutrition for proper healing.

It's very important that you complete your postoperative exercises and walk as soon as possible after your surgery to assist your bowels in returning to normal function. Sometimes, despite all of your efforts, you will still experience some abdominal bloating and discomfort. Not only is this very uncomfortable but it can put a strain on your abdominal *sutures* (stitches). Inform your nurse of the problem and she will speak with your physician so that your bowel problem can be addressed as soon as possible. It may be necessary to give you medication or an enema to stimulate your bowels.

Postoperative Complications

No one likes to think they will suffer complications after their surgery. However, sometimes complications do occur as a result of the surgery, your primary disease, or other factors. Complications may include problems with the surgical incision, lung problems, *urinary retention* (temporary inability to urinate), blood clots, and infection. Lung complications and blood clots can usually be avoided by faithfully following instructions for your postoperative exercises. The following exercises should always be approved by your doctor and nurse before you begin doing them. We have included a checklist to make it easy for you to keep track of how many times you do each approved exercise every day. Keep the checklist and a pencil next to your bed.

Breathing Exercises to Prevent Pneumonia

Immediately after your surgery, the nurses in the PACU (recovery room) will ask you to take some deep breaths. This is necessary because while you were lying asleep on the operating room table your breathing was assisted by the ventilating equipment. You were not taking the normal breaths that fully expand your lungs and keep them inflated and free of fluid.

On the nursing unit, your nurse may instruct you in postoperative exercises for deep breathing and coughing. These may seem ridiculously simple, but they are very important. Deep breathing and coughing help to fully inflate your lungs with air, increase your blood circulation, and prevent the accumulation of secretions or mucus in the air passages. If you don't clear your lungs of these extra secretions, they will build up and lead to pneumonia.

Sometimes you will be given a simple tool that is called an *incentive spirometry* or *triflow unit* to use during your breathing exercises. This is a small plastic box with three chambers. Inside each chamber is a pingpong ball. You will be instructed to inhale deeply through a mouth piece, raise the pingpong balls inside the chambers to a certain level, and then hold them in this raised position for a few seconds. This allows you to see how effective your deep breathing is and encourages you to make steady improvement so that you prevent lung complications. Ask the nursing staff or respiratory therapist to explain how you should use the triflow (also called an inspirometer) since various models may work differently.

For the most part, they work in the following manner:

1. Hold the plastic box upright. It's important that it is not tilted.

2. Exhale, then seal your lips around the mouthpiece.

3. Take a deep, slow breath until the balls all rise midway
    or higher. Keep the balls raised by holding your breath
    for a count of three.

4. Remove the mouthpiece and exhale normally. Rest a
    minute, taking several normal breaths. Then repeat
    using the inspirometer, raising the balls each time. Do
    this at least 10 times every two hours that you're awake.
    It may be best to avoid using the inspirometer immedi-
    ately before or after meals (it may cause nausea).

It's very important that you make a conscious effort to
continue using your triflow unit or take deep breaths and cough
every two hours throughout your recovery period. This includes
the time you are recovering at home.

Next are some suggested guidelines for breathing and
coughing exercises. Review them with your physician or nurse
and, if they approve, do these every two hours, or more often
if appropriate.

Deep-Breathing Exercise

1. Sit on the edge of your bed or in a chair with your legs
    dangling down from the knees. Or lie in bed with your
    head propped up on pillows. The object is to be in an
    almost full sitting position .

2. Gently exhale slowly and completely.

3. Inhale with a slow, deep breath, breathing through your
    nose. If you breathe through your mouth you may swal-
    low air that will give you gas. You should be able to feel

your chest expand if you have taken a deep
enough breath.

4. Hold your breath and count to five, then exhale slowly
    and completely through pursed (puckered) lips. You
    should feel your chest deflate.

5. Repeat this exercise five times, always concentrating on
    deep breaths that fully expand your lungs.

6. Take a fourth deep breath. As you exhale, give a forceful
    cough. Your incision cannot be opened by coughing, but
    the act of coughing tugs and pulls on the incision, mak-
    ing it hurt. If you have had the type of surgery where
    this causes discomfort (for example, abdominal surgery)
    it may help to protect your incision by holding a pillow
    snugly against your abdomen or to place one hand on
    each side of your incision and hold the incision area
    together to decrease discomfort.

7. Repeat this coughing exercise at least three times fol-
    lowing your deep breathing exercises. Take short rest
    periods between each cough.

You may find that you cough out a great deal of mucous
during this exercise, so have plenty of tissues handy. Coughing
exercises are important to do postoperatively, especially if you
are elderly, have a history of lung problems, such as asthma,
bronchitis, or emphysema, or are a smoker. Deep coughing helps
to loosen and mobilize secretions that have accumulated in your
lungs while you were lying on the OR table.

Generally, the only time you should avoid coughing is if you
have had certain ear or eye surgeries, have had a large abdominal

hernia repaired, or have had brain or throat surgery. In these special cases, or when advised to avoid coughing by your nurse or physician, you will only do deep breathing. If during your preoperative evaluation your nurse does not instruct you on coughing exercises, ask if your particular procedure is one that restricts the use of coughing exercises.

You will need to do these breathing exercises and coughing even when it hurts. Remember, it's normal to have some discomfort following surgery. Your muscles may ache or feel strained from lying on the hard operating room table, or you may have pain in the area where the surgeon made the incision because your skin and muscles were cut which caused nerve irritation.

You will be tempted to favor the area of your surgery. You may be reluctant to sit up straight, take deep breaths, and cough because it causes pain. If you let this temporary discomfort prevent you from deep breathing, coughing, and walking you risk developing *pneumonia.*

It's important that you take your pain medication so that you are able to move about and prevent further complications like pneumonia. The best plan is to take your pain medication, wait 15 or 20 minutes until it takes effect, then do your breathing exercises. Rest a few minutes, then ask your nurse if you may go for your walk or do the other exercises that have been suggested by your physician, nurse, or therapist.

Leg Exercises to Prevent Blood Vessel Inflammation and Clots

The following leg exercises will help you prevent *thrombophlebitis* (inflammation of the blood vessels and possible formation of blood clots) after surgery. These exercises are also good if

you have been ill for some time prior to surgery and have had
your normal daily activities limited, have a history of poor circulation in your lower legs, or have had surgery on your legs, your
abdomen or your heart.

The purpose of these exercises is two-fold. First, they help
increase the blood flow to your lower legs. As your leg muscles
contract and relax, the working muscles massage the smaller
blood vessels in the lower leg and increase the flow of blood
through the veins. Second, these exercises help maintain
your muscle tone which allows you to get up and walk soon
after surgery.

You may find that these exercises are more strenuous than
you expected to do after surgery. Take your time and pace yourself. Do not strain excessively. Also, make certain these exercises
have been approved by your physician and nurse before starting
the program.

Leg Exercise

1. While lying in bed on your back with your legs comfort-
    ably outstretched, bend your right knee and put the sole
    of your foot flat on the bed.

2. Lift your lower leg off the bed by raising your foot until
    it is even (parallel) to your knee. This is a slow, gentle
    movement, like kicking an imaginary football.

3. Lower your foot back to the bed.

4. Repeat this exercise five times. Next do the same with
    your left leg.

Foot & Ankle Exercise

1. While lying in bed on your back with your legs comfortably outstretched, lift your right foot a few inches off the bed.

2. Rotate your ankle in a complete circle five times, then rest your foot on the bed for a moment.

3. Raise your foot off the bed a few inches. Point your toes toward the foot of the bed then point your toes toward the head of the bed. Do this foot stretch five times.

4. Repeat with your left foot.

Thigh and Calf Exercise

1. While lying in bed on your back with your legs comfortably outstretched, tighten your thigh muscles then relax. Repeat this five times with each leg.

Turning in Bed

If you will be confined to your bed for the first day or so after your surgery, it's helpful to know how to turn yourself in bed. This is especially true if you have had some type of abdominal surgery—although you may not normally be aware of it, we use our abdominal muscles to roll from side to side and to sit up. If you're feeling too uncomfortable to turn, that is a sign indicating that you are not taking enough pain medication.

There are several reasons why you should change position in bed at least every two hours:

- The muscle movement increases your blood circulation.
- It promotes better respirations by taking pressure off one side of your chest and allowing your ribs to fully expand.
- It allows the blood to circulate to your skin and prevents pressure sores (bed sores) from forming due to decreased circulation to the areas you are lying on.

All too frequently, elderly patients lie in one position too long and the circulation to their tissue is decreased to the point that the skin becomes reddened and eventually breaks down into an ulcerated area. This can happen much quicker than you realize, so move about as much as you can.

How to Minimize the Discomfort of Turning in Bed

1. Lower the head of your bed so that your mattress is flat.

2. If you had abdominal surgery, hold a small pillow against your abdomen.

3. Have the nurse raise and lock, in an upright position, the bedrail on the side of the bed you wish to turn toward. If you want to turn to the right, raise the rail on the right hand side of the bed.

4. Bend your knee on the opposite side of the direction in which you wish to turn and place your foot flat on the bed. If you want to turn to the right, this will mean your left foot is flat on the bed.

5. Reach over and grab the side rail with your hand that is closest to the railing while holding the pillow to your abdomen with the other hand. If you are turning right,

grab the right rail with your right hand and hold the pillow with your left hand.

6. Roll over in one smooth motion by pulling on the siderail and pushing off with your bent knee and foot at the same time.

Once you are on your side, you may find that it increases your comfort to have the nurse place one pillow between your knees and ankles and wedge another pillow tightly against your back to provide support. The head of your bed can now be raised slightly until you feel comfortable. Remind those who are caring for you to relocate your call light, TV control, light control, and bedside table to the side of the bed you have been turned to face.

DAILY POSTOPERATIVE EXERCISE CHECKLIST   DATE: _____

INSPIROMETER (ENTER TIME)	DEEP BREATHING AND COUGHING	LEG EXERCISE	FOOT AND ANKLE EXERCISE	THIGH AND CALF EXERCISE

CHAPTER TWELVE

Medications in the Hospital and at Home

Scenario

In the past your need for medication was limited to a few aspirin for an occasional headache. Your current medical condition requires many medications, taken several times a day. Although you trust your physician and agree that the medication has helped relieve some of your symptoms, every time you swallow another pill you wonder if there is any information you should have beyond the instructions the pharmacist gave you when she filled your prescriptions.

We think there are some important points about medications that every patient should know in order to be safely medicated. This chapter will discuss them in a question and answer format so that you may skip any areas with which you are already familiar.

What are medications? Do they differ from drugs or pharmaceuticals?

In general usage, the terms have the same meaning: a chemical or substance given to a patient to *aid in the diagnosis of disease, prevent or treat disease, heal injuries* or *relieve pain and discomfort.* The study of drugs or medications is called *pharmacology* which is why persons educated to prepare and dispense drugs (or medications) are called *pharmacists.* The place where a pharmacist does his or her business is the pharmacy. We often interchange the terms and call the pharmacy a drug store and the pharmacist a druggist. Another term for a pharmacy, not in common usage today, is *apothecary.*

185

How are medications administered?

There are several routes by which a medication can be given to a patient. The patient's age, symptoms, overall condition, and medical history, as well as the desired effect of the drug and the chemical composition of the drug often dictate the preferred route. The major routes are *oral* (put a pill, liquid,or capsule in the mouth and swallow it); *topical* (apply to the surface of the skin); *sublingual* (place beneath the tongue to dissolve); *rectal* (insert into the rectum); and *parenteral* (use a needle to inject directly into tissue or into the blood stream via a vein). Many drugs can be given in a variety of routes. Your physician will decide upon the best route for you.

What is the difference between a local and a systemic drug?

Local drugs are administered to a chosen site on the body where they exert an effect limited to that specific area. Examples of this are ointments applied to skin that is inflamed from an encounter with poison ivy or medication gargled for a sore throat. *Systemic* drugs are administered at one site in the body but then enter the bloodstream and are distributed throughout the body. An example of a systemic drug is penicillin. It can be administered as pills that are swallowed, dissolved in the stomach and then absorbed into the bloodstream (oral), or it can be given by injection into a muscle and then absorbed and distributed (parenteral). The route of administration differs, but because it affects the whole body, it is considered a systemic drug.

Why do some medications require frequent doses?

One of the body's techniques for maintaining a healthy state is to rid itself of foreign substances (*detoxification*). The body perceives medications as foreign material and diligently works to eliminate them. This detoxification process is carried out by the liver, kidneys, and the lungs, with a majority of drugs processed and eliminated by the liver, a significant number by the kidneys, and a small number by the lungs. How efficient the body is, and how long the drug can exert its effect, give each drug an individual time schedule. The *time of onset* (when the drug begins to work), the *peak effect* (when the drug is working at its maximum strength), and the *duration of action* (how long the drug exerts an effect) are known for each drug. In order to maintain a consistent therapeutic dose in the body, drugs are administered so that an even effect is achieved. It's important to keep in mind that the liver, kidneys, and lungs can be damaged if a medication is taken in too high a dose or more frequently than recommended. Liver or kidney failure caused by drugs is rare if drugs are taken according to the physician's directions. The idea of "if one is good two are better" definitely does not apply to medications.

What is the difference between the over-the-counter drugs and prescription drugs?

Over-the-counter drugs are available for purchase without a physician's written order (*prescription*). They will treat the symptoms of minor diseases and injuries that do not normally require you to seek a physician's care. For example, these medications are used to treat headaches, constipation, muscular aches, indigestion, colds, and flu. Generally, they are safe if taken as directed on the container label. Prescription drugs must be ordered by a licensed physician or dentist and prepared and dispensed by a licensed pharmacist. Prescription drugs can be very powerful and must be used according to your physician's instructions. Their effects are carefully monitored by your physician to be certain they are safe and effective.

A prescription drug will be identified by the symbol Rx on the physician's written order and sometimes on the container's label. Examples of prescription drugs include antibiotics, narcotics, and steroids. Some drugs that are at one time sold only as prescription drugs eventually become available over-the-counter, although often in a weaker strength (for example, Motrin).

How does a generic drug differ from a brand-name drug?

The ingredients in a generic drug and a brand-name (or trade name) drug are theoretically identical. The federal government has regulations to ensure that all the products sold as medication dissolve and can be absorbed into the bloodstream. The difference is that the generics are sold under the name of the active chemical ingredient rather than the trade name given to that chemical by the pharmaceutical company. Assigning a trade name is simply better marketing because it is much easier for people to remember a brand name. An example of a trade or brand name is Tylenol whose generic name is *acetaminophen*. The trade name products are patented for a number of years by the pharmaceutical company that developed them. The companies tend to try and recover their research and development costs by charging more for the medication while it's under patent and they are the only supplier. Once the patent expires, other companies can manufacture the same medication, but since they don't have research costs to recoup, they will sell it at a lower price. In some cases, the generic drug can be significantly less expensive than the trade name drug (20 to 800 percent less). When generics become available, the brand-name price will often decrease in response to this new competition.

If generic and trade name are the same, why do some people think the generic drug is not as effective for them as the trade name?

The Food and Drug Association (FDA) rates drugs and also performs dose equivalency tests to determine if medications are equal. However, although the drugs rate as equivalent ,there are some other factors to consider. Even when rated the same, the generic may have different inactive ingredients which produce a different level of medication in the bloodstream. This makes it necessary to adjust the dose. An example is Tegretol™, an anti-seizure drug. The brand-name and generic versions of Tegretol™ are *bio-equivalent*, but if the patient is switched from one to the other, the dose must be adjusted to account for the way each version is dissolved and absorbed into the bloodstream. Patients may also experience what is termed the *placebo effect*. This is a situation in which the patient's expectations of a medication actually influence the experienced effect. For example, if you always take Bayer aspirin because you think it is the most effective, and then purchase a generic aspirin you doubt will be as good, it may not be as effective for you.

Should I be concerned about medications purchased in foreign countries?

The FDA has jurisdiction over the safety and efficacy of medications approved for use within this country only. There is no way to know what medications purchased in other countries contain. The ingredients, as well as the methods for manufacturing the medication may differ. Obviously, different ingredients may change the effect of the drug, but the manufacturing process is also important. For example, if a tablet or capsule is compressed too tightly, it will literally pass all the way through the body and never dissolve to be absorbed into the bloodstream.

What are drug side effects and contraindications?

Side effects of medications are undesired actions of a drug. It may simply be that the desired effect of the medication is greater than anticipated, or that other effects not directly related to the action of the drug appear. Side effects can sometimes be controlled by adjusting the dose or the method and timing of administration. For example, if a drug causes nausea, taking it with food may be recommended. Other times a different drug will have to be substituted for the first prescription. *Contraindications* are reasons not to give the drug or to discontinue it. Contraindications may include allergy to the drug, pregnancy, and pre-existing liver or kidney disease.

How will I know if I'm allergic to a drug?

The allergic response in the body requires at least one exposure to the drug (or a very similar drug) before it reacts abnormally to a dose of medication. Unfortunately, the only way to know if you have an allergy to a medication is if you have a reaction after taking it. These reactions can range from a minor skin irritation, to nausea and vomiting, to life-threatening anaphylaxis (extremely low blood pressure and difficulty breathing). The allergic response can become more serious with repeated exposures to the offending drug. If you have even a mild reaction (for example, a skin rash) to a medication you will want to inform your physician before taking additional doses. It is also *extremely important* that you discuss any known medication allergies with your physician. Some drugs are very similar in chemical structure and if you are allergic to one you may be allergic to another drug in the same "family." As an example, let's say a patient takes a few doses of penicillin and develops nausea, wheezing, and a skin rash on his chest and arms. If he continues taking the penicillin he risks progressing to an anaphylactic reaction, so his physician discontinues the penicillin and gives him another antibiotic that is unrelated to penicillin. A year later the patient seeks care from a new physician and neglects to tell her about his penicillin rash. The new physician prescribes a cephalosporin which, although not actually penicillin, is closely related to penicillin. The patient takes one dose of the cephalosporin and has an anaphylactic reaction.

Is it safe to share medications?

No. Medications are prescribed specifically for you. Your physician has taken into account your age, weight, overall condition, medical history, signs and symptoms, medication history, and allergic history. You should **never** share medications with another individual because there are too many differences among individuals and disease states. Don't take anyone else's medication and don't give yours to anyone else.

Is it safe to adjust the dose of medication myself if what the doctor ordered does not seem to be effective?

No. Again, your physician has ordered what he or she thinks is the best dose for you. If you think the dosage needs adjusting, or if you wish to discontinue taking it, discuss your situation with your physician. Remember, too much medication may harm your liver and kidneys, and too little may not be therapeutic.

Do I always have to continue taking my medication, even if I feel better?

This is a question to ask your physician if you feel better and want to stop taking your medications. Generally, the amount of medication and duration of therapy prescribed is best for your situation and should be followed. Some medications, such as pain medications, may be prescribed to be taken "only as needed" for relief of pain. If you are not uncomfortable, you may not need the pain medication. On the other hand, antibiotics must be taken for a full course in order to guarantee that all of the *microorganisms* causing your disease are dead. Sporadically taking antibiotics may allow the germs to develop a resistance to the antibiotic, compounding your problems. Remember, when prescribing medications your physician takes into account your individual history and the drug's peak action, duration of action, and desired effect.

Are there any combinations of medications, foods or alcohol that I should avoid?

Medications can cause an unwanted reaction and be harmful if taken together, with certain foods, or with alcohol. To help prevent these interactions, it is very important to inform your physcian about *all* the medications you are currently taking, even common over-the-counter drugs like cold medicine. If you drink wine, beer, or spirits, discuss your drinking habits with your physician. It is often very dangerous to mix medicines with alcohol.

How long can I keep medications?

It is very tempting to keep left-over medications "just in case" you need them again. However, outdated products can decompose and become dangerous, causing severe reactions. You should not use any medication beyond the expiration date on the label. This is true for both prescription and over-the-counter drugs. Dispose of them safely. Many people dump outdated medications into the toilet and flush.

Where is the best place to store my medications?

Most people store their medications in the worst place in the house: the bathroom cabinet. Every drug is unique, but many are sensitive to heat and moisture. The warmth and moisture from the shower or bath can cause medications to decompose and change. Likewise, carrying medications in a pocket, leaving them in the car's glove compartment or carrying them in a back-pack exposes them to heat which hastens their breakdown. If the medications have been left in a hot place for an extended period of time (a month or longer) it's best to check with the pharmacist to see if that specific medication is adversely affected by heat. Try to store medication containers in a cool, dry, dark place that is out of the reach of children, such as in an empty shoebox on a bedroom closet shelf or in a drawer. If you must carry medications with you, carry only what you need while you are away from home. When traveling by commercial airplane, never pack them in checked luggage because lost luggage may take several days to catch up with you. It's best to keep medications in their original containers as much as possible to allow easy access to identification, instructions, and expiration dates. **Never** switch a medication to another, different medication container or mix several medications in a single container. Not only do you risk becoming confused over which pill is what medication, but if providers need to identify your medications in an emergency, the jumbled pile of pills is a difficult puzzle to sort out.

What can I do to keep track of my medications and remind myself to take them?

There are several products available in many drug stores or by mail order that serve as medication dispensers and reminders. Some are simply plastic boxes with the days of the week on them. Others will set off an alarm at a preset time, and so forth. Which device you purchase depends upon how much memory jogging you need. Many patients find marking a calendar or homemade checklist sufficient. If you must take multiple medications and prefer not to purchase a pill organizer, an empty cardboard egg carton can be marked with the correct days or times and your medications counted out in each appropriate egg indentation. If you keep your medications in their original containers, you may find it helpful to mark the tops with colored dots designating different times of the day (for example, red for 8 a.m., blue for 9 a.m. and 9 p.m., green for bedtime, etc.) Try to get your medications on a schedule that synchronizes as many of the doses as possible, after clarifying with your physician or pharmacist that the drugs may be taken together. For example, if medication A is to be taken every six hours and medication B is to be taken at bedtime, arrange it so that one of A's six-hour doses coincides with your bedtime. That would be A at 10 a.m., 4 p.m., 10 p.m. and 4 a.m. with B at 10 p.m. also. Space your doses out according to your physician's instructions, but set the schedule to your lifestyle.

Does it make any difference where I purchase my medications?

Where you buy your medications is very dependent upon the type of health insurance coverage you have. It may be that your insurance plan will only pay for prescriptions filled by a particular pharmacy or through certain mail-order houses. If you are able to fill your prescription in several pharmacies, call ahead and ask for a price quote. Some large chains may offer you a better price. In terms of *discharge medications* ("take home" or medications you take home after hospitalization), most inpatient insurance companies will not pay for discharge medications. You may find it most cost effective to get only a few days supply of medications from the hospital pharmacy to tide you over until you can get the remainder of the prescription at a pharmacy your insurance will cover. If you want this option, ask your physician to write a prescription for a few days' worth to be filled in the hospital pharmacy and another larger prescription for the outside pharmacy. If a medication is prescribed during an office visit to your physician, she can sometimes provide you with a few free samples. These samples will supply you with medication until you can get your prescription filled. Physician-supplied samples may be especially helpful if you are concerned about tolerating the medication, will be on it a very short time, or will be tapering off a medication. The pharmacy is not able to take back unused medications or exchange them for a newly prescribed drug. Whatever amount of medication you purchase is yours. Mail-order pharmacies (for example, those available through AARP) are usually less expensive and may be the best option for you, especially if you will be taking the same medication for an extended period of time.

Is all medication packaged the same?

No. Most pharmacists will package medications in a child-proof container unless you specifically request otherwise. If you have difficulty opening the childproof tops, ask for the easy open top that flips off. If you have trouble reading the small print on the container, ask for larger type or written instructions in larger type. If your medications are packaged in "blister packs" that you find difficult to open, ask for the pills to be poured into a container. Always read the label and make certain that it lists your name, the correct drug, and the correct strength. Read the instructions and make certain you understand them. Check the expiration date. Read all the warning stickers and make certain you understand them.

Questions to ask about your medications (ask your physician and/or pharmacist)

- What is the name, type, and prescribed dose of medication?

- What is the purpose of taking it? (why was it prescribed?)

- How long will I be taking the medication? (days/weeks/months/years?)

- How do I take the medication (by what route?)

- Are there special administration techniques? (for instance, is there a special way to place eye drops into the eye? Do I need to shake liquids thoroughly?)

- When do I take the medication? (times? with food? as needed?)

- Are there foods or drinks I should avoid while taking this medication? (for example, cheese or alcohol, etc.?)

- Are there any activities I should avoid while taking this medication? (driving, operating machinery, etc.)

- What should I do if I forget a dose?

- Are there side effects I should watch for? What are they?

- What should I do if I think I'm having side effects?

- Are there special storage requirements? (refrigeration? darkness?)

- Are printed instructions and drug information available for me to take home?

MEDICATIONS AND ALLERGIES LIST FOR: _____ *your name*

MEDICATION	STRENGTH	DOSE	HOW OFTEN	LAST DOSE	WHY TAKEN	SPECIAL INSTRUCTIONS

If you are allergic to any medications, products or foods, please list them and briefly describe what type of reaction they cause. For example, penicillin gives you a rash or peanuts make you wheeze, decongestants make you nervous, or adhesive tape burns your skin.

MEDICATION/PRODUCT/FOOD	REACTION

CHAPTER THIRTEEN

Discharge: Going Home and Home Health Care

Scenario

During your physician's evening visit to your hospital bedside he tells you that he has written your discharge orders and that you will be going home in the morning. While you are delighted that your hospital stay is almost over, you are also nervous about going home. You know you are still too weak or disabled to tolerate leaving your house, and that you need continued medical care and assistance. Perhaps you will require tube feedings at home. You may be struggling with bathing and dressing yourself. You need to learn how to move into a sitting position in your own bed, and you are uncertain how to pay for the special equipment you need to walk. Suddenly you (or your loved ones) feel very unprepared to manage your care at home. What should you do?

Home Health Care Services

It is very important that you, or your loved ones, share your concerns with your physician and nurse. In most cases, you have a nurse discharge planner/utilization coordinator or case manager assigned to you. This individual has been evaluating your readiness to go home and the types of support services, if any, you will need. She or your physician may have reviewed your case and may have already begun the process of arranging your health care services at home. It is always wise, however, to say you are worried about needing help at home and to ask what resources are available to provide it. While it is most common for the staff or physician to initiate home care services, you and your family also have the right to ask for home care.

There are many types of help available from a variety of medical professionals and nonmedical staff for patients who need support and/or treatment in their homes. Inhome therapeutic medical services include skilled nursing services, medical social services, physical therapy, occupational therapy, speech therapy, and nursing assistant (home health aide) services. Additionally, nonmedical staff can provide housekeeping and meal preparation services. All of these services are often collectively called "home health care" or "home care." The purpose of home care is to provide you and your family and/or care givers with the support necessary to allow you to remain at home and still safely and successfully manage your health care needs.

Home care is not to be confused with hospice care, although hospice care can be provided in your home. Hospice care is basic medical care and pain relief for terminally ill people who have a physician's prognosis of less than six months to live. Hospice care provides the patient and family with counseling, support, and an environment free from high-technology life-sustaining interventions. The goal is to allow the patient to die with dignity, surrounded by loved ones. (For information on hospice care contact: National Hospice Organization, 1901 North Moore Street, Suite 901, Alexandria, VA 22209. Telephone: 800-658-8898)

The organization that employs home care medical professionals/staff and coordinates their services is called the home health care agency. Some agencies will offer a limited number of services while others, such as the Visiting Nurses Association, are full-service agencies and offer the entire spectrum of services. Home health agencies can also be a hospital department, affiliated with a hospital, a community not-for-profit organization, or a private for-profit company.

The need for home care is frequently determined by your diagnosis. There are some diagnoses that almost always require follow-up home visits: total joint replacement; newly diagnosed diabetes; and chronic obstructive lung disease requiring lung drainage and oxygen. Other medical situations are not so clear cut for justifying home care: after chemotherapy, or recovering from a heart attack. Criteria for helping your physician decide whether or not you need home care includes the following:

- Your age
- Your degree of independence
- Whether you will be home alone or with a care giver
- Your care giver's or family's ability to provide support
- Where you live (remote versus in-town and near resources)
- What kind of treatments you need (wound care, teaching, or emotional support)
- If you have required home care in the past

If your physician decides you need home care, he may order several different types of services immediately. Alternatively, he may request a home care nurse to visit you in your home to assess your situation and determine what specific services you will benefit from most. The type and recommended frequency of visits is discussed with you and your caregivers, then individualized to your situation and payor's guidelines.

Your home care nurse will call you at home to arrange this first visit. It's very helpful if you have a calendar available to avoid scheduling conflicts with your other appointments and activities. It's also most efficient if you have written out the directions to your house so you can clearly read them to her.

The nurse and any other professionals involved in your care will each write a plan of care and treatment goals with your input and collaboration. Any changes to your plans will be discussed with you, your caregivers, and your physician. Remember, home care is a *partnership* between you, your caregivers, and the home care service providers. Your ongoing, active participation is very important.

When your physician orders home care for you, how much of the cost will be covered by your insurance is determined by each individual insurance company or payor. Medicare and Medicaid have stringent criteria for determining if you are eligible for home care and which services they are willing to pay for. For example, the basic home care eligibility requirements for Medicare are:

1) A physician's order authorizing home care
2) A need for part-time or intermittent skilled care
3) A medically reasonable and necessary need for treatment
4) That the patient be "home bound." The federal government provides the home health care agencies with several guidelines for determining if a patient is truly home bound. Some federal indicators for home-bound status include:
   - restricted mobility from disease process
   - poor cardiac reserve, shortness of breath, or activity intolerance due to a worsening disease process
   - bed– or wheelchair–bound patients who require physical assistance to move any distance

- a patient who requires caregiver help with a cane, walker, wheelchair, etc.
- failure to thrive, low birthweight infants
- a tracheostomy, abdominal drains, foley catheter, or other tubes that restrict walking
- inability to walk with portable oxygen, home ventilator dependence
- confusion, impaired mental status, or psychosis that restricts ability to function outside the home
- fluctuating blood pressures or blood sugars that cause dizziness
- inability to use stairs or walk on uneven surfaces without help
- eye surgery and physician-ordered activity restrictions
- being legally blind or unable to drive
- natural disasters or geographic barriers that make it very difficult for patient to leave the home

Private insurance companies and HMOs each have their own set of eligibility criteria. Regardless of their criteria, keep in mind that in most cases they require that your physician justify the need for home care and write an order for the services. Equally important is for you to determine that the agency providing your services is a state licensed and federally certified home health care agency in order to bill your insurance company. Many insurance companies will only pay for services provided by a licensed and/or certified home health care agency. The following resources can help you determine if your agency is licensed and certified:

1) your state, county, or local department of health and human services. (Actual department names vary slightly from state to state, and are listed in the telephone directory under "Government.")

2) National Association for Home Care
   519 C Street, N.E.
   Washington, DC 20002
   202-547-7424

3) Foundation for Hospice and Home Care
   519 C Street, N.E.
   Washington, DC 20002
   202-547-6586

Even in cases when eligibility is uncertain, most insurance companies will pay for at least one home visit after discharge from the hospital to evaluate the patient, the home environment, and the social situation. During this evaluation visit (most frequently conducted by a home care nurse) your ability to function independently, your or your caregiver's ability to meet your healthcare needs, and the physical safety of your home are all assessed.

If, after the evaluation, it is determined that you do not meet your payor's criteria for home care, you may still independently call an agency and request to privately purchase home care services. In this case, it is especially important that you purchase only those services you need. The hospital social worker or discharge planner may also be able to provide you with the names and telephone numbers of other community resources such as Meals-on-Wheels, private physical therapists, vendors of medical equipment, transportation agencies, and Senior Centers or Area Agencies on Aging, as appropriate.

Once you have attained the goals outlined in your plan of care, or it is determined that you no longer need or qualify for home care, you will be discharged from the home care services. Your home care providers will discuss this with you prior to terminating your home visits.

If, at any time, you have complaints about your home care services, the agency should have provided you with a "hot line" telephone number to call to register your complaints or concerns. Failing a satisfactory response from the agency, your state or county Department of Health and Human Services will have a consumer complaint telephone number to call. This number can be found in the telephone directory under "Government."

"Home Alone" Without Home Health Care Services

In some instances you will not need home health care services, or you will choose to decline them. This does not mean you are completely without any help or resources. If you have had an outpatient procedure you will not be sent home until your vital signs are stable, you are able to stand and walk without dizziness and nausea, your pain is controlled or alleviated, you are able to urinate, you know who you are, where you are and why you are where you are, and you show an understanding of your postoperative instructions. These same guidelines often apply to patients who have spent an overnight or more in the hospital following a surgical procedure.

Your nurse will review your postoperative instruction with you and your caregivers. She will advise you to watch for any unusual drainage from your surgical wound (for example, bright red blood, green, yellow, or foul-smelling discharge, sudden and large amount of any fluids soaking your bandages); red and "angry" looking sutures or closures; a spreading area of red, warm skin surrounding your incision; a new opening in your incision; or new and unrelieved pain. She will ask you to be certain you are drinking fluids and urinating, and that you are able to move your bowels within the next few days (return of bowel movements may vary depending upon your diet and type of procedure, so check with your nurse).

The nurse or pharmacist will review the name, purpose, dose, and timing of any medications. Be certain you have this information in writing. Refer to the previous chapter on medications for hints on scheduling and managing your medications.

All of the deep breathing, coughing, and leg/ankle exercises discussed in Chapter 11 are still important for you to continue at home. It may be tempting to crawl into the comfort of your own bed or recliner and just sleep, but resist the temptation. Ask your caregiver to wake you, or set an alarm and get up and walk around the house for several minutes every two or three hours during the day. This is also the perfect time to do your breathing and leg exercise to promote your circulation, improve your lung function, and help get your bowels back on schedule.

It's also a good time to remind yourself that the procedure is now behind you, and to visualize yourself once again enjoying life as a healed and healthy individual. There are several self-help books and relaxation tapes available at local bookstores and libraries. You may find the visualization exercises and guided relaxation techniques helpful as you recover. If your surgery was the result of a serious disease or condition, there may be support groups in your community where people with similar experiences can help you as you recover. The Internet also has chat rooms for people in similar situations who enjoy participating in electronic conversations.

While you were in the hospital eating institutional food you may have thought a big juicy hamburger or vegetarian pizza was exactly what you were going to eat for your first meal at home. We caution you to consider what type of foods you were eating and tolerating in the hospital, and not to jump too quickly to rich, heavy, or spicy foods. Remember, to avoid nausea, bloating, and abdominal cramps, you want to progress from ice chips to clear liquids to soft foods to a regular diet. Some patients find it helpful to start with small, frequent meals and then gradually return to a regular meal portion and time. Don't forget to drink several glasses of water or other clear fluids throughout the course of the day. Again, frequent small sips may be easier to tolerate than drinking an entire glass of apple juice at once.

You are never truly without resources, even when you are recovering at home alone. Your physician will either be available "on-call" himself, or will have designated another physician to answer incoming calls from patients. A call to his office will reach either his front office staff during business hours or his answering service after hours and at lunch time. If you think your concern is urgent, it is important to convey that information to the person answering the telephone. Call back time may vary from a few minutes to a few hours to a few days unless you are very specific about why you are calling. If you are having severe pain, shortness of breath, dizziness, bleeding, etc., you must tell the person exactly what those symptoms are and how long you have had them. Many physicians have advice nurses who can offer you excellent advice and support. Some insurance companies also employ advice nurses who will answer your questions about symptoms or other healthcare issues.

If you received your care at a teaching hospital, someone will be on-call for the group of doctors or "service" responsible for your care. It is helpful for the hospital operator if you ask for whomever is covering your attending physician's service. So, if the *attending physician* (most senior faculty physician on your team) was Dr. Milliken, ask for whomever is covering Dr. Milliken's service. One of the residents will return your call.

Failing a response from anyone, you always have the option to call the local emergency department. They will probably advise you to come into the ED to be seen, because they do not know you or your case. This is not the most efficient way to get help, but if you truly think your case is urgent or an emergency, you should not hesitate to call them, dial 911 or call an ambulance.

PREOPERATIVE TASKS CHECKLIST FOR

_____
Your name and social security number

INSURANCE:

Name of insurance company:_____

Plan type and number: _____

Insurance company telephone number:_____

Full name of representative spoken with: _____

Date/time of conversation:_____

INFORMATION YOU MAY NEED FOR DISCUSSION WITH INSURANCE COMPANY REPRESENTATIVE:

Your employer:_____

Work area code and telephone #: _____

Your primary care MD's name: _____

_____   _____
         address   *telephone*

Your surgeon's name: _____

_____   _____
         address   *telephone*

Surgical procedure: _____

Date/time of surgery: _____

Place of surgery: _____

_____   _____
         address   *telephone*

DOCUMENT THE FOLLOWING ADDITIONAL INFORMATION:

Summary of covered services:
  Hospital
  Physician
  Laboratory/X-Ray

Summary of charges you will be responsible for:

Additional comments:

ADMITTING PAPERWORK:

Your address: _____

| number | street | apartment # |

_____

| city | state | zip |

Your telephone number : _____

Insurance company and plan
(see card if available): _____

Birthdate: _____

Social security number: _____

Place of employment: _____

ADDITIONAL DOCUMENTS TO CONSIDER:

❑ Consents _____
❑ Living will _____
❑ Do not resuscitate _____
❑ Patient Bill of Rights _____
❑ Organ donations _____

PHYSICAL EXAMINATION:

Date: _____

Time: _____

Place: _____

Parking instructions: _____

_____

Special instructions: _____

_____

Previous surgeries and dates: _____

_____

Blood replacement preferences: _____

Instructions to donate blood: _____

_____

Questions about your surgery or recovery: _____

_____

Instructions for:
- ☐ Deep breathing exercises
- ☐ Diet
- ☐ Medication /Allergies List
  (see provided form)

CHAPTER FOURTEEN

When You're Feeling Better

Scenario

The surgery was successful. You're recovering nicely in the comfort of your own home. Your anxiety about the whole experience has long since faded, and you're looking forward to resuming your normal activities. Then, into the relative calm of this post-surgery period comes something guaranteed to send your blood pressure soaring and your nerves jangling ... the bill.

Impossible to understand, laden with mistakes and overcharges — that's the commonly held perception of hospital bills. Unfortunately, the perception is all too often correct. The fact is, there is a strong likelihood that your bill will contain at least one — or possibly many — errors. As for being impossible to understand, the average person may find Sanskrit more comprehensible than the typical itemized hospital bill.

If the prospect of months of befuddlement, helplessness, and wrangling with your hospital, physician, or insurer over potential billing errors is not an appealing one, take heart. A savvy patient can take charge of the situation and minimize the time and stress involved in paying their hospital bill and resolving any billing disputes. When it comes to your hospital bill, fiscal and emotional mayhem need not be your destiny.

The Prevalence of Billing Errors

Just how prevalent are hospital billing errors? National studies have demonstrated that anywhere from 90 to 97 percent of all hospital bills contain inaccuracies — and, of course, these miscalculations are rarely in the patient's favor.

This pervasive billing problem has enormous implications for the health care system as a whole. By some estimates, hospital overcharges may account for as much as $28 billion in health care costs every year. Insurers who routinely pay hospital overcharges must recoup their expenses by raising premiums, causing health care costs to continue to spiral out of control. In the end, everyone pays.

Meanwhile, these billing errors extract a tremendous personal toll as well. Individuals may spend many frustrating months, or even years, trying to resolve billing problems, which can ultimately wreak havoc on their credit and financial well-being.

Why are so many hospital errors being made? When you consider the sheer complexity of a typical hospital stay which involves the integration of dozens or perhaps hundreds of individuals from many different departments, each of whom must log every aspect and expenditure of your care, from a single dose of aspirin to a transfusion, and then submit them for central compilation (along with those of every other patient in their care) billing errors are, if not forgivable, then at least understandable. Just a single mistake in coding—which is generally done by hand—can result in thousands of dollars in errors in a single bill.

Clearly, when it comes to hospital bills, patient vigilance has never been more important.

A Little Advance Planning

Some of the most important things you can do to mitigate potential problems and ensure a streamlined insurance reimbursement process should be done before your surgery.

First, study your insurance manual and make sure you thoroughly understand your medical coverage. Do not simply depend on your health care provider to know your benefits. If you are undergoing an elective procedure that your policy does not cover, you will certainly be in for a rude awakening — and no recourse other than to pay out of your own pocketbook — when the bill comes. If you are covered by Medicare, which is always subject to revisions, call your local office to make sure that you have an up-to-date overview of benefits. The same applies to any supplemental medical insurance (medigap) policy you might have.

While you're reviewing your insurance benefits, don't forget to check the expiration date of your policy. Make certain that your coverage will not lapse during treatment or postoperative recovery period. Pay any pending premiums in a timely manner.

Assuming that your pending surgery is covered by your insurance policy, it's essential that you (or your physician's office) obtain the proper authorization(s) for the procedure before entering the hospital. If the physician who performs the initial procedure should refer you on for another procedure, you should not depend on that referring physician to obtain an approval for the next procedure. Remember that an authorization applies only to the specific procedure or visit requested, not for the entire course of treatment, unless that is the normal pathway for that particular treatment. For example, if you're coming in for a cardiac biopsy, one would normally have certain testing and lab work done in conjunction with that procedure. Therefore, approval for the cardiac biopsy should theoretically include these items. However, if during the course of that biopsy another medical problem is identified which requires a different set of tests, those separate services would not be covered by the original authorization, and you would need to obtain a second one.

Some institutions have financial counselors to assist patients in determining any special insurance requirements and obtaining the necessary pre-authorizations prior to surgery. Additionally, they may be able to give you a rough estimate of charges before you enter the hospital so there are no surprises when the bill comes.

Good Notekeeping

Once you've obtained an authorization from your insurer, keep a record of the authorization number(s), as well as the name of the person providing the number, the date, time, etc. Good notekeeping can make all the difference later when it come time to unravel your bill.

While you're in the hospital, it's also an excellent idea to keep a detailed diary of your stay. If necessary, enlist the aid of a family member or friend to help you document specific procedures, tests, or any special services or equipment that you use or receive while in the hospital. Keep track of medications (what they are and when you receive them), I.V.s, injections, changes of dressing,and anything else that seems pertinent. Later, when the bill arrives, it will be that much easier to determine the validity of specific charges if you can rely on a detailed log rather than your memory.

Your surgeon or the nurse or manager in the operating room can review the portion of the bill allocated to your operating room experience.

When Can I Expect To Receive a Bill?

Every institution has a different billing system, and timetables for getting a final bill to the patient will vary accordingly. Generally, patients will not receive a bill until after their insurer has been billed and has remitted payment for the appropriate portion of the covered charges. The hospital then bills the patient for any remaining balance, which becomes known as the "patient's responsibility."

In some cases, especially if you are undergoing an elective, ambulatory procedure at a freestanding surgical center, you might actually be handed a bill on the way out the door. Never pay a bill on the spot unless you've agreed in advance to pay a specific amount, which is accurately reflected on the bill. You will need time to thoroughly review the charges, and the hours after one emerges from anesthesia are certainly not the best time to tackle a detailed medical bill. If you do need more time, insist on taking the bill home with you. Do not let the cashier pressure you into paying prematurely.

Given the turnaround time required for insurance reimbursement and back-and-forth documentation, it's more likely that you will receive a bill anywhere from two weeks to several months after surgery. It's not completely unheard of, however, to receive a bill as late as a year after the procedure. Waiting for that bill can in itself be a source of frustration and anxiety, especially when you're trying to do accurate financial planning.

Before you receive your actual bill, you might be sent an interim statement from the hospital indicating the total charges that have been billed to your insurer. Additionally, your insurer may send you a statement detailing the amount they have paid to the hospital, and the amount that is the patient's responsibility. Be certain to save these insurance statements so you can later check them against the reimbursement amounts on your hospital bill; this is a potential area for mistakes.

Be aware that your initial hospital bill may not include charges for the physicians who participated in your care (surgeon, assistant surgeon, radiologist, anesthesiologist, etc.) You may receive a separate bill (or possibly multiple bills) for these fees. Not infrequently, patients are taken completely by surprise when an eye-popping second invoice arrives after the first bill has been cleared up.

Making Sure Your Bill is Correct

Always demand an itemized bill. This is the most important step you can take to protect yourself from billing errors. Do not simply accept a bill that shows only the amount your insurer has paid, and the amount for which you are responsible. In this era of managed care, itemized bills may be going the way of the starched white nurse's cap, but, as asserted in the Patient's Bill of Rights (discussed in Chapter 7) every patient is entitled to a full examination and explanation of the hospital bill.

Your itemized bill will probably contain many pages of charges — everything from doses of aspirin to laboratory work to CT scans. Most bills are full of abbreviations, and many charges may be simply bundled under the category "Miscellaneous." As daunting and as byzantine as this document may seem, you need to spend some time analyzing it. A few minutes of your time can result in significant savings to you and your insurer, so it's important to read the statement carefully.

You may notice that your hospital bill or insurance statement contains certain items or services that have been "discounted." These discounted items are based on the contract that each insurer has drawn up with your health care provider.

Start With the Basics

Check your name. (And even if the first page is correct, make sure that some other patient's pages haven't been stapled to your bill by mistake, something that has been known to happen.)

Check the dates of your hospital stay against those on the bill. Are you being billed for the correct number of days?

Make sure you're being billed for the correct kind of room (private, semiprivate, etc.) If you had a bed in a short-stay surgical unit, which some hospitals are now offering at reduced cost, make sure that the appropriate room rate has been applied.

If you spent any portion of your hospital stay in an intensive care unit (ICU), coronary care unit (CCU), make sure that the correct number of days has been allocated to each, because the per diem charges are much higher for these specialized units than for the conventional "med-surg" beds.

The More Complicated Part

Review each line item and make certain that you actually received the tests, procedures, supplies, medications, etc. outlined in the bill. Did you actually undergo that CT scan, X-ray, or lab test? Refer back to your hospital log to check on any dressings, injections, etc. that you may have received, or any supplies, such as crutches, support devices, humidifiers, thermometers, etc., and make sure that no unrequested or unused items appear on your bill.

Do the charges for preadmission testing accurately reflect the workup you received? The hospital may have automatically charged you a set fee covering a full battery of preoperative tests, when you did not actually require or receive all those tests.

Look especially hard at any medications for which you're being billed, because this can be a prime area for mistakes. For instance, you may have been erroneously charged for a daily dose of a certain medication, when in fact you only received it on the first day of your stay.

Look for any duplicate charges, particularly if you received services on both an inpatient and outpatient basis.

If You Find a Billing Error

If you identify any problems with your bill, there are several approaches you can take to resolving the problem. The best place to start is usually the hospital billing department (sometimes called Patient Financial Services, or by a similar name), since they are the closest to the problem and can quickly identify the departments or individuals that generated the disputed amount(s).

Another possible avenue open to you is to contact the representative within the human resources or benefits department at your place of employment (if you obtain your coverage through your job). Some employers actually pay a reward to employees who manage to identify hospital errors that result in savings to the company.

You can also call your insurance company directly. If you're calling to report a hospital overcharge, you may be surprised to find that they are less than enthusiastic about pursuing an error, even if it means that the reimbursement to your health care provider was too high. The insurer may feel that the overcharge was not significant enough to be worth devoting personnel to auditing the bill.

Finally, if your procedure was done at a freestanding clinic or physician's office, there may be a dedicated contracts or HMO person on staff who can help you resolve the problem.

Whatever you decide, do not start out by calling every conceivable person at once. Not only will it result in unnecessary duplication of effort, but the situation will only get more confusing if multiple people at multiple places are working on the problem at the same time. Also, resist the temptation to dash off a letter to the hospital CEO. This should be viewed as an option of last resort, to be used only after you have exhausted all conventional problem-solving channels.

In the rare event that you feel the overcharges in your bill represent an intentional criminal act by your hospital, you should contact the office of the state attorney general.

If the problem with the bill relates to denial of insurance benefits rather than errors or overcharges, you and the hospital will need to work with your insurer to make sure that the proper documentation has been provided. Patients with Medicare should always exercise their right to appeal if payment for certain services has been denied.

Presenting Your Case

In many cases, the billing error can be cleared up with a single phone call, particularly if it's a question of a readily identifiable error, such as a single mistake in coding, or a CT scan billed in error. If the situation is more complex — or has become that way due to multiple rounds with the hospital and your insurance company — you may want to request a face-to-face meeting with a billing department representative.

Bring along a record of the insurance authorization number(s) you received prior to your surgery and the names of all insurance representatives you spoke with, as well as a copy of your "explanation of insurance benefits," to your meeting.

It may be difficult, but try to be as patient and remain as calm as possible when explaining your problem. You do not want to put the billing representative on the defensive, or begin the relationship in an adversarial manner. You may be dealing with this person for some months to come, and it's far more beneficial to you if they are an ally.

At the end of the meeting, make sure that the individual fully understands the problem. Ask for an estimate of how long it will take to resolve the error, and what actions they will need to take. Finally, be sure to establish what the next steps will be. When can you expect to hear back from the person with some kind of status report? Will they phone you directly? Will you receive something in writing? Let them know that you will phone them on such-and-such a date to check back in if you have not heard anything.

It's always a good idea to follow up by sending a written summary of the discussion to your billing representative. You can copy the department billing manager on this correspondence.

(You might wish to prepare this written summary of the problem in advance and bring it to the meeting.) When putting the problem in writing, remember the most important rule: stick to the pertinent facts. Be concise. No one has the time nor the desire to wade through a 20-page document recounting every conceivable detail of your case. You do not need to let them know that you arrived at 5:30 a.m. for the operation, accompanied by your mother and cousin Sadie. Include just enough details to identify the case, the issues that are in dispute, and the history of the dispute resolution. To make your history as easy to follow as possible, try using bullet points or presenting the information in outline form.

If the billing representative has estimated that it will take two weeks to resolve the problem, wait at least that long before contacting them again. As with any similar situation, while you want to be persistent, you certainly don't want to end up being viewed as a pest.

You should always try to work with the same people in the benefits or billing office when trying to unravel a problem. However, if there is a slow response — or no response at all — to your initial meeting or follow-up calls, contact the billing department manager.

How Long Should Bill Resolution Take?

Every organization and problem is different, so it is difficult to predict how long it will take to resolve your particular billing problem. In some cases, problems can be resolved within 24 hours.

If an appeal needs to be made to the insurance company, documentation needs to be gathered, which means that the process could take several months.

If there are multiple insurance companies involved, it could take from seven to eight months to a full year for the paperwork to be exchanged, reviewed, audited, and verification made prior to the patient receiving a bill.

Methods of Last Resort

Suppose you've had umpteen rounds of communication with the hospital and the insurance company, and the problem remains unresolved. Perhaps the hospital is refusing to admit its mistake. Or perhaps you've been promised a credit, but months have gone by and you're still waiting for that credit to be applied to close out your account. Meanwhile, the collection agency is starting to call and your credit has been compromised. It's time to apply the methods of last resort.

If you've been dealing with a specific representative within the billing department for the entire time, contact the manager of the billing department. You may have to go over the person's head as well. If this fails to produce expedient results, then it's time to involve the hospital chief executive officer.

Depending on the nature of the problem and the hospital's attitude, you may also need to call an attorney and initiate legal proceedings.

If all else fails — and you don't mind being a feature segments on the evening news — some local television stations will step in and become advocates for people attempting to resolve thorny medical billing problems. This is a long-shot, of course — you're competing for attention with landlord/tenant disputes, auto mechanic scams, and the like — but if you have a particularly irksome problem that remains unresolved after months of good-faith attempts to get justice, a local reporter and camera crew can sometimes help get your case the attention it requires. Similarly, newspapers in some cities offer action line columns to bring problem-solving assistance to readers.

Filing a Complaint With the State

If you believe your insurer has failed to act in good faith by denying all or parts of your medical claim, and all resolution attempts have failed, you can file a complaint with the state insurance department.

Your complaint must be in writing, and contain the following information:

- Your name, address, and telephone number
- The name, address, and telephone number of your insurance company
- Pertinent information about your policy, including identification number, type of policy, etc.
- The reason for filing your complaints

Paying Your Bill

Maybe you actually received a completely accurate bill from the start. Or you've gone through several rounds of error resolution, your insurer has made payment, and you finally have a total that you believe is correct. That means it's time to pay that bill.

Different issues and problems may now be at stake. Patients who are underinsured or uninsured may be unable to pay the outstanding balance immediately. Some insured patients may find themselves with a higher balance than they anticipated.

Patients who have difficulty paying their bills in full can negotiate with the hospital to develop a payment plan. Generally, hospitals want most bills paid in six months. Different hospitals will use different criteria for handling aging accounts or unpaid balances, including when and if your account will be reported to credit bureaus. Most hospitals will allow 90 - 120 days from the point at which the bill becomes the patient's responsibility (for example, after all insurance payments have been made.) Generally the first notice goes out in 30 days, a second in 60 days, and a third at the 90-day point.

If a patient has not paid the bill by this point, or at least made payment arrangements, the hospital may elect to send the bill to a collection agency. Collection agencies charge interest and receive a percentage of the charges collected. If a patient decides to initiate contact with the hospital after a unpaid bill has gone for collections, they will likely be told to resolve the problem directly with the collection agency.

Be aware that once you have racked up a bad debt at a hospital you may not be able to return to that hospital for future treatment.

Appreciation and Acknowledgment

Now that you're feeling better, there's one more thing to take care of before you close the chapter on your surgical experience. Think back on your hospital stay, and all the individuals who participated in your care. Reflect on all the things that were positive about your stay ... and any that weren't.

Then, write a few thank-you notes to express your appreciation to the key individuals involved in your care, and to anyone else who performed some extraordinary service for you or your family. Start with a note to your surgeon. To acknowledge the many nurses who provided care for you, you can address a group note to the head nurse (or "nurse manager") and ask them to post it for all to see. Were there any other individuals (for example a physical therapist) who worked closely with you, or any patient relations representatives, administrators, pastoral care representatives, etc. who went out of their way for you or your family? Don't forget about any personnel who helped you resolve a billing problem.

Be as specific as you can in these letters of appreciation. Let each individual know what they are doing right or wrong. Not only are most caregivers delighted to receive such letters of acknowledgment, but your comments can be invaluable in helping to improve service for all the patients about to embark on their own surgical experience.

RESOURCE INFORMATION

1. 800-23-ERROR, a telephone number to report often unreported hospital mistakes.

2. Board of registered nurses for each state. You can find your local telephone number by calling the American Nurses Association. (202) 651-7000.

3. Medicare information:
   Health Care Financing Administration, Department of Health and Human Services, 200 Independent Avenue, SW, Washington, D.C. 20201. Oversees Medicare programs. 800-772-1213.

4. Medicare Publications, HCFA Inquires
   6325 Security Blvd., Baltimore, MD 21207
   Medicare Handbook, 1996
   Guide to Health Insurance for People with Medicare
   Medicine and Advance Directives

5. Medicare Hotline
   Department of Health and Human Services
   800-638-6833

6. Social Security Administration
   Department of Health and Health Services
   6401 Security Blvd., Room 4J5, West High Rise
   Baltimore, MD 21235.
   (301) 965-1234
   800-772-1213

GLOSSARY

ASA 1–ASA 5: *Categories of patients defined in terms of their risk for surgery by the American Society of Anesthesiologists. ASA 1 being the lowest-risk patient.*

Abdominal drains: *Soft plastic or latex tube placed in the surgical site to drain excess fluids.*

Acetaminophen: *The generic name for Tylenol.*

Advance directives: *Forms for a living will and a durable power of attorney.*

Allopathic hospitals: *Traditional hospitals, where disease and injury are treated with medical and/or surgical interventions.*

Ambulatory: *The ability to walk.*

Amnesia: *Memory loss.*

Analgesic: *Pain-relieving medication.*

Anaphylactic shock: *The most severe form of allergic reaction, resulting in vascular collapse and coughing.*

Anesthetic agents: *Medications used to relieve pain, sedate, and relax a patient during surgery. Anesthetic gases include Halothane, Forane, or some agents mixed with nitrous oxide.*

Aneurysm: *A weakened, bulging area in a blood vessel.*

Anesthesia: *General or localized inability to feel pain, caused by drugs or "numbing" agents used during surgery or other painful procedures.*

Antibiotics: *Medications such as penicillin, gentamicin, and sulfas used to kill bacteria that cause illness or infection.*

Anti-emetic: *A drug given to prevent or relieve nausea and vomiting.*

Anti-inflammatories: *Medications used to decrease swelling, redness, and pain. These may include aspirin, Motrin, or Naposin.*

Aspirin: *An anti-inflammatory available over the counter.*

Appendicitis: *An inflammation of the appendix.*

Arbitration: *The hearing or determination of a dispute between parties by a person chosen or agreed to by them.**

Arthroscopy: *Use of an endoscope for the diagnosis or surgical treatment of diseased or injured joints.*

Attending physician: *At a teaching hospital, the most senior faculty physician on the medical team.*

BP: *Blood pressure.*

BSO: *See bilateral salpingo-oophorectomy.*

Bair hugger: *A temperature-controlled blanket used to add warm air over a surgery patient*

Barbiturates: *Any of a group of barbituric acid derivatives, used in medicine as sedatives and hypnotics. **

Battery: *Offensive or injurious physical contact. In the world of medicine, this term can be applied to giving care or performing procedures without a patient's informed consent.*

Benzodiazepenes: *A group of drugs (Librium, Valium, Xanax, and Ativan) used to relieve anxiety and during conscious sedation to enhance amnesia.*

Bio-equivalent: *Medications — either generic or brand-name — that are almost identical chemically, and have the same effect on the body.*

Bilateral salpingo-oophorectomy (BSO): *Removal of the ovaries and Fallopian tubes, parts of the female reproductive tract necessary for normal conception.*

Biopsy: *Removal of tissue from the body for microscopic examination to aid in determining diagnosis.*

Blood pressure cuff: *A soft cloth monitoring device for blood pressure.*

Body temperature: *The heat produced by the body's metabolism balanced against the heat lost from the body's surface. Normal adult oral temperature is 98.6 degrees Fahrenheit.*

Brachial plexus block: *Anesthetic used in surgery for carpal tunnel syndrome.*

Bunionectomy: *The surgical removal of a bunion.*

Carpal tunnel syndrome: *A disorder of the hand characterized by pain, weakness, and numbness in the thumb and other fingers, caused by an inflamed ligament that presses on a nerve in the wrist.**

CCU: *Coronary care unit.*

CNA: *Certified nursing assistant, aide, or orderly.*

Capitated: *A system used by HMOs in which the primary care physician is compensated with a fixed amount of money for patient care.*

233

Case rate: *A flat amount paid to hospitals by Medicare.*

Cephalosporin: *Any of a group of widely used broad-spectrum antibiotics, derived from the fungus Cephalosporium acremonium.* *

Chaplaincy: *Priests, ministers, rabbis, or trained lay people available on call to contribute to the healing process by providing spiritual counsel and emotional support in a hospital environment.*

Cholecystectomy: *Removal of the gall bladder and accompanying stones.*

Chronic: *An ongoing medical condition.*

Chronic hypertension: *Blood pressure that measures 140/90 or higher when checked in a series of readings.*

Clinical social worker: *A professional who can counsel a patient and family as well as provide practical support to help cope with the effects of illness or hospitalization.*

Codeine: *A pain medication.*

Coinsurance: *Insurance underwritten jointly with another insurer. (or, a percentage of the total bill.)* *

Community hospitals: *Hospitals serving a particular area or community.*

Conscious anesthesia: *Anesthesia that blocks pain without loss of consciousness. The patient remains awake, breathes normally, but does not feel pain. In some cases the patient will not remember the operation.*

Contraindication: *Reason not to give a drug to a patient, or reasons to discontinue a drug. These may include allergy, pregnancy, and pre-existing liver or kidney disease.*

Copayment: *A flat fee charged to the buyer of health insurance for various medical services.*

Contaminants: *Bacteria, fungus, virus, other foreign materials that make an area dirty or unsterile.*

Craniofacial surgery: *Surgery performed to the head or face.*

DRG: *Diagnosis related group. A patient classification system that associates a patient diagnosis to the cost incurred by the hospital. DRGs are used as a basis for prospective payment or reimbursement.*

D. O.: *Doctor of Osteopathic Medicine.*

Darvon: *A pain medication.*

Deductible: *The amount for which the insured is liable for each claim made on an insurance policy.**

Demerol: *A pain medication.*

Detoxification: *The body ridding itself of foreign substances in order to maintain a healthy state.*

Diagnostic dyes: *Dyes injected into the body to help a physician visualize and evaluate organs and vessels.*

Diastolic pressure: *The lower number in a blood pressure reading (generally 60-80 in a healthy adult).*

Dilaudid: *A pain medication.*

Discharge medications: *Medications a patient takes home after hospitalization, also known as take-home medications.*

Do not resuscitate order: *An order coming from a physician directing the hospital and nursing staff about what should not be done in the event the patient stops breathing and/or their heart stops beating.*

Draping: Positioning several sterile towels around an incision site in preparation for an operation.

Durable power of attorney: A legal document in which a competent adult gives another competent adult the right to make his or her health care decisions, including the refusal of life-sustaining treatments, should the person writing the durable power of attorney become unable to make decisions.

Duration of action: How long a drug exerts an effect.

EKG/ECG: Electrocardiograms.

Elective surgery: A surgical procedure that can be performed at the patient's convenience and is the patient's choice.

Electroencephalographic: Using an instrument for measuring and recording the electrical activity of the brain.*

Electrocardiogram: The graphic record produced by the electrical activity of the beating heart.

Electrolytes: Ions or elements in the body, including potassium, calcium, and magnesium, that are essential to life.

Emergent surgery: Surgery performed for a life-threatening condition or one that may rapidly worsen until it causes serious damage or cripples the patient.

Emesis basin: A basin used to collect vomit.

Endoscopy: Using a hollow tubular instrument to measure the interior of a body cavity or hollow organ.*

Enema: The introduction of a fluid into the rectum for treatment or cleansing of the bowels.

Epidural anesthetic: *An anesthetic agent injected into the area around the spinal cord to block pain sensation to the abdomen or lower extremities. Frequently used during Caesarean section for childbirth.*

Epidural blood patch: *Procedure in which patient's blood is used to stop a cerebral spinal fluid leak.*

Exclusion: *A provision in an insurance policy that denies certain coverage.*

Fentanyl: *An anesthetic drug.*

Flatus: *Gas.*

Foley catheter: *Soft rubber tube inserted into the bladder via the urethra to drain urine.*

For-profit: *A hospital that is in business to make a profit.*

Free-standing surgery center: *A surgery center in a location separate from a hospital, such as a high-rise or elsewhere.*

Gatekeeper: *Primary care physician who monitors and approves a patient's medical care by the HMO.*

General hospitals: *Most hospitals are general hospitals, usually providing medical, surgical, and diagnostic services under one roof, with designated wards for similar types of patients.*

Gentamicin: *An antibiotic.*

Group insurance: *An insurance plan under which a number of persons and their dependents are insured under a single policy, issued to their employer or to an association with which they are affiliated, with individual certificates given to each insured person.* **

HMO: *Health maintenance organization.*

Hematocrit: *A measurement of packed red blood cell volume, expressed as a percentage of the total blood volume.*

Hemoglobin: *The compound attached to red blood cells that carries oxygen to the body's tissues and carbon dioxide away from the tissues.*

Hernia repair: *An operation to repair the protrusion of an organ or tissue through an opening in its surrounding walls, especially in the abdominal region.*

Hospice care: *Basic medical care and pain relief for people who are terminally ill, with a prognosis of less than six months to live.*

Hospital-based ambulatory surgery center: *A surgery center that is located within the hospital buildings, providing no overnight stays; patients must be stable to use this center.*

Hypertension: *Abnormally high blood pressure.*

Hypotension: *Abnormally low blood pressure.*

Hysterectomy: *Removal of the uterus.*

ICU: *Intensive care unit.*

Implied consent: *When it is inferred that the patient consents to whatever treatment is necessary for life-saving and health preservation.*

In vitro fertilization: *Assisted reproductive technique where a woman's ripe eggs are surgically removed, fertilized in the laboratory, and the pre-embryo replaced into her uterus.*

IPA: *Independent practice association.*

I.V.: An intravenous line. Plastic tubing attached to a needle and inserted into the middle of a patient's vein. Sterile solution is run through the vein, and it becomes a passage for the administration of medication.

Incentive spirometry/triflow unit: Also called an inspirometer. A tool used during breathing exercises to measure the efficiency of deep breathing.

Intra-arterial line: Plastic tubing inserted into an artery.

Informed consent process: A process by which the person performing treatment or an operation on a patient must provide complete information about the procedure to the patient and obtain the patient's consent to perform the procedure before beginning it.

Inpatient unit: The part of the hospital devoted to overnight or long-term patients.

Insurance authorization: When a patient's insurance company authorizes a medical procedure.

Intraoperative stay: Time spent in surgery.

Invasive: When equipment must be inserted into the body.

JCAHO: Joint Commission on Accreditation of Health Care Organizations. This organization monitors patient-centered performance standards and accredits a hospital facility accordingly.

Johnny gown: A hospital gown.

LVN: Licensed vocational nurse.

Laboratory technician: A phlebotomist. This person obtains blood samples when the physician orders tests on blood content.

Laparoscopy: A procedure used to look inside the body using a tiny, metal scope the size of a drinking straw.

Living will: A living will states specifically which life-sustaining measures a patient permits or refuses. It is effective while the person is alive and has nothing to do with the type of will leaving property to a person's heirs after death.

Local anesthestic: An anesthetic that is given to block pain only in the surgical region. The patient is aware of what is going on during surgery, but cannot feel pain.

Local drug: A drug that is administered to, and remains at, a chosen site.

Major blood types: A, B, AB, and O denote genetically determined substances (antigens) on the surface of the red blood cells.

Managed care: Health plans that have financial incentives in place to control costs.

Mastectomy: Removal of the breast.

Medical centers: Very large general hospital offering the latest in technology and using the most recent medical findings.

Medical emergency: A serious health condition that threatens life or limb.

Microorganisms: Any organism too small to be viewed by the naked eye, such as bacteria.

Motrin: An anti-inflammatory pain medication.

Morphine: A narcotic and pain medication.

NCQA: National Committee for Quality Assurance.

Narcotic: *Any of a class of habituating or addictive substances that blunt the senses and, in increasing doses, cause confusion, stupor, coma, and death. Some are used in medicine to relieve intractable pain or induce anesthesia.* *

Neurological check: *Evaluation of a patient's brain and spinal cord function, including assessment of mental status, function of cranial nerves, and other reflexes.*

Neurosurgical: *Surgery involving the brain or other nerve tissue.*

Non-invasive: *A procedure that does not require entering the body.*

Not-for-profit: *An institution that does not exist to make a profit, but simply to cover operating expenses.*

Novocain: *A numbing medicine often used by dentists.*

Numbing medicines: *These include Novocain and xylocaine.*

Nuprin: *An anti-inflammatory.*

Occupational therapist: *A professional who can help a patient develop or adapt skills to regain physical independence following illness or surgery. This includes daily living activities, such as dressing, eating, and personal care.*

Office-based surgery: *Surgery performed outside of a hospital in a physician's office; usually less costly to the patient.*

Open enrollment: *An annual opportunity offered through an employer to an employee to enroll in a new health plan or switch from one plan to another.*

Oral: *Given to a patient by mouth.*

Oral airway: *A plastic device that keeps the tongue from falling into the back of the throat and closing off the airway during surgery.*

Osteopathy: *A system of medical practice emphasizing the manipulation of muscles and bones to promote structural integrity and relief of certain disorders.**

Osteopathic hospitals: *Hospitals staffed primarily by doctors of osteopathic medicine.*

PACU: *Post anesthesia care unit or recovery room.*

PCP: *Primary care physician, such as an internist, family practitioner, or general practitioner. Often referred to as a gatekeeper since a patient must go through this physician to ensure that medical care is paid for by the HMO.*

POS: *Point-of-service programs.*

PPOs: *Preferred provider organizations (see below).*

PCA: *Pain control machine; specialized medical equipment that allows the patient to self-medicate to relieve pain.*

Pain medications: *Drugs used to relieve or prevent suffering. Examples include morphine, codeine, and aspirin.*

Paralytic ilius: *When bowels stop their normal function in reaction to the trauma of surgery.*

Parenteral: *A medication that is given by injection.*

Patient assessment unit; Preoperative testing unit; Preadmission testing unit; Preoperative anesthesia clinic; Preoperative assessment program; Preoperative processing: *Various names for a special area for evaluating patients who are scheduled for surgery.*

Patient autonomy: *The American health care system recognizes this as the patient's right to independence, freedom, and self-determination. The right to consent to or refuse treatment.*

Patient Bill of Rights: *A bill of rights that has been approved by national and statewide hospital organizations, medical societies, nursing organizations, etc., describing a patient's rights regarding health care. For example, care must be given without regard to race, sex, ethnicity, religion, or source of payment.*

Patient Self-determination Act: *Federal legislation passed in 1990 requiring all hospitals and health care agencies receiving Medicaid or Medicare funds to advise patients about their right to consent to and/or refuse treatment, and about the availability of advance directives such as a living will or durable power of attorney.*

Peak effect: *When a drug is working at maximum strength.*

Pediatric: *The branch of medicine concerned with the development, care, and diseases of babies and children.**

Penicillin: *An antibiotic.*

Pharmacist: *A person educated to dispense drugs or medications.*

Pharmacology: *The study of drugs and medications.*

Pharmacy: *The place where a pharmacist does business. It used to be called an apothecary.*

Pharmacy services: *The hospital department staffed by licensed pharmacists, with expertise on medications.*

Physical therapist: *A professional who develops exercise therapy personalized for the patient both during and after a hospital stay to help strengthen muscles and teach a patient how to move on crutches or a walker, etc.*

Placebo effect: *A situation in which the patient's expectations actually influence the experienced effect of an inactive "sugar pill" or other inactive substance.*

Pneumonia: *Inflammation of the lungs with congestion.**

Preadmission paperwork: *The filling out of forms by a patient preceding admission into a hospital or clinic for surgery.*

Preferred providers: *A preferred provider organization (PPO) has contracts with a large network of physicians, hospitals and other health providers at discounted rates. When a member of a PPO uses their services most of the bill is paid by the managed care plan.*

Premium: *Monthly fee paid to cover insurance cost.*

Preoperative examination: *A physical examination administered to a patient preceding an operation or procedure to ensure that the person is healthy enough to undergo surgery.*

Prescription: *A doctor's order for a medication or drug.*

Private hospitals: *The most common type of hospitals in the U.S. Many operate as nonprofit businesses and receive their funding from private sources such as local physicians or universities, or from government funds, such as hospital bonds.*

Prophylactically: *As a precaution. When a medication or device used to prevent a specific condition, it is said to be given prophylactically.*

Propofol: *A drug administered during surgery by an anesthesiologist to render the patient unconscious.*

Postoperative: *Following an operation.*

Pulse: *The regular throbbing of the arteries, caused by the successive contractions of the heart, especially as may be felt at an artery, such as at the wrist.**

Pulse oximeter: *A device used to measure the oxygen content of the blood.*

Public hospitals: *These include those managed by a city, county, public health service, or the military. Many public hospitals serve society's poor.*

Rh factor: *A person's blood is either positive or negative for this substance. Rh is short for Rhesus monkey, the mammal in which this factor was first identified.*

RN: *Registered nurse. This person has passed a licensing test and has extensive knowledge of pathophysiology and nursing science.*

Radical dissection: *A major surgical procedure that results in extensive loss or restructuring of tissues.*

Radiology technician: *The person who takes a patient's X-rays.*

Regional anesthesia: *Anesthetics used for certain types of surgeries to block specific regions of the body, for example, epidurals.*

Respirations: *The exchange of oxygen and carbon dioxide during the movement of air in and out of the lungs. Each rise and fall of the chest counts as one respiration. Evaluated for rate, rhythm, and volume of air exchanged per minute.*

Respiratory support: *Assisted breathing via a mask or ventilator.*

Respiratory therapist: *A professional who helps a patient maintain adequate lung function. This person assists patients with coughing or deep breathing exercises, and helps them use respiratory machines, as needed to keep lungs inflated and clear.*

Rotator cuff tear: *Injury to any of the four small muscles that hold the bones of the shoulder in position.*

Scrubs: *Simple cotton uniforms worn by medical personnel working in surgery.*

Sedation: *Relaxation or sleep.*

Sedative: *A drug or agent that soothes or sedates.*

Serum: *Clear liquid in the blood.*

Short-stay unit: *A hospital ward for patients who will not be there longer than 24 hours.*

Sodium pentothal: *A sedating agent.*

Specialty hospital: *A hospital providing services to only one type of patient, for example, women or children only.*

Splinting: *Using a rigid material to hold a bone or any part of the body in position.*

Staff HMO: *An organized prepaid health care system delivering health services through a salaried physician group employed by the HMO. Kaiser is the most famous staff model HMO.*

Step-down PACU/phase II PACU: *An area of the PACU unit where same-day surgery patients who are planning to go home are assisted in going to the bathroom and dressing.*

Stethoscope: *An instrument used in auscultation to detect sounds in the chest or other parts of the body.**

Sublingual: *Medication that is melted under the tongue.*

Suction catheter: *Soft tube attached to a vacuum pump used to suction fluids out of the body. For example: to suction excess fluid out of the mouth.*

Sulfas: *Antibiotics.*

Sutures: *Stitches.*

Systemic drug: *A drug administered at one site of the body that spreads throughout the entire body.*

Systolic pressure: *The higher number in a blood-pressure reading (generally 95-140 in a healthy adult).*

TPR: *Temperature, pulse, respirations—the vital signs for life.*

Teaching hospitals: *Hospitals that also serve as sites for educating students. Often, patients must interact with the students in teaching hospitals.*

Talwin: *A pain medication.*

Thrombophlebitis: *Inflammation of the blood vessels and possible formation of blood clots.*

Time of onset: *When a drug begins to work.*

Tonsillectomy: *Surgery for removal of the tonsils.*

Topical: *A medication or drug given by applying it onto the skin.*

Tracheostomy: *The construction of an artificial opening through the neck into the trachea, usually for the relief of difficulty in breathing.**

Urgent surgery: *A surgery procedure that must be performed within the next 12-24 hours.*

Urinalysis: *Chemical analysis of urine. These are actually several tests done on the sample provided.*

Urinary catheter: *A tube inserted into the bladder to drain urine.*

Urinary retention: *The temporary inability to urinate.*

Valium: *A tranquilizer.*

V.A., or Veteran's Administration hospitals: *These are either specialty hospitals (for example, psychiatric hospitals) or general hospitals which limit their patient population to members or veterans of the armed services or their dependents.*

Vital signs: *The vital processes necessary for life, including breathing, blood pressure, etc.*

White coat hypertension: *A rise in blood pressure experienced only when the patient is in the presence of a physician.*

Xylocaine: *A numbing medicine.*

*Random House Webster's College Dictionary, New York: Random House, 1991.

**Sharing the Risk, published by the Insurance Information Institute, 3rd ed. New York, 1989.

REFERENCES

Books

Baker, R. *Successful Surgery: A Doctor's Mind-Body Guide to Help You Through Surgery.* Old Tappan, NJ: Pocket Books, Co. 1996.

Bruno, P., Craven, R., Patrick, M., Rolosky, J., Woods, S. *Medical-Surgical Nursing: Pathological Concepts.* 2nd ed. Philadelphia: J.B. Lippincott Co., 1991.

Buzby, G.P., Mullen, J.L. "Nutrition and the Surgical Patient." In Goldman D.R., Brown F.H., Levy, W.K., Slap, G.B., Sussman, E.J., eds. *Medical Care of the Surgical Patient.* Philadelphia: J.B. Lippincott, 1982.

Covino, B.G., Scott, D.B. *Handbook of Epidural Anesthesia and Analgesia.* New York: Greene & Stratton, 1985.

Deardorff, W., Reeves, J. *Preparing for Surgery: A Mind-body Approach to Enhance Health and Recovery.* Oakland, CA.: New Harbinger, Co., 1997.

Drain, C.B., Christop, S.S. *The Recovery Room.* Philadelphia: W.B. Saunders, 1987.

Earnst, F.W., Pace, W., Frederich. *Now They Lay Me Down to Sleep: What you don't know about anesthesia and surgery can hurt you.* W. Earnst, Co., 1997.

Hahn, A.B., Oestreich, S.J.K., Barkin, R.L. *Mosby's Pharmacology in Nursing.* 16th ed. St. Louis: CV Mosby, 1987.

Hall, Jr., C.P. "Hospital Plans," *The Handbook of Employee Benefits: Design, Funding, and Administration,* 2nd ed., Rosenbloom, J.S., ed. Homewood, IL.: Dow Jones-Irwin, 1989.

Hicks, Stallmeyer, Coleman. *The Role of the Nurse in Managed Care*. Washington, D.C.: American Nurses Publishing Co., 1993.

Huddleston, O., Northrup, C. *Prepare for Surgery, Heal Faster: A Guide by Mind-body Techniques*. Cambridge, MA.: Angel River Press, Co.,1996.

Inlander, Charles B. *150 Ways to be a Savvy Medical Consumer*. Allentown, PA.: The People's Medical Society Co., 1992.

Inlander, Charles B., Weiner, eds. *Take This Book to the Hospital with You: A Consumer Guide to Surviving Your Hospital Stay*. Allentown, PA.: The People's Medical Society Co., 1993.

Keating, Karen. *Take Charge of your Hospital Stay: A "Start Smart" Guide for Patients and Care Partners*. New York: Insight Books, 1994.

Lemone P., Burke, K. *Medical Surgical Nursing: Critical Thinking in Client Care*. Menlo Park, CA.: Addison-Wesley, Co., 1996.

Macho, J., Cable, G. *Everyone's Guide to Outpatient Surgery*. Kansas City, MO.: Andrews and McMeel, Co., 1994.

McConnell, E.A:*Clinical Considerations in Perioperative Nursing*. Philadelphia: J.B. Lippincott, Co. 1987.

Merenback, Lisa. *Working with Capitation: The Advanced Training for Operating Room Clinical Specialties Modules*. Cypress, CA.: Medcom, Inc., MHSA Co.,1995.

Phippin, Mark, Wells, Maryann Papanier. *Perioperative Nursing Practice*. Philadelphia: W.B. Saunders, 1994.

Rice, Robyn, R.N., M.S.N. *Home Health Nursing Practice: Concepts and Application*. St. Louis, MO.: Mosby, 1996.

Rongstvedt, P.R. *The Managed Health Care Handbook*. Rockville, MD.: Aspen Systems Co., 1989.

Shimberg, E., Blau, S. *How to Get out of the Hospital Alive: A Guide to Patient Power.* Old Tappan, NJ.: MacMillan, 1998.

Smith, C.E. *Patient Education.* Orlando, FL.: Grune & Stratton Co., 1987.

Snow, J.C. *Manual of Anesthesia.* 2nd ed. Boston: Little, Brown & Co., 1982.

Sobel, D.S., and R. Ornstein.*The Healthy Mind, Healthy Body Handbook.* Los Altos, CA, 1996

Vickey, D., Fries, J. *Take Care of Yourself: A Consumer's Guide to Medical Care.* Menlo Park, CA.: Addison-Wesley Publishing Co., 1978.

Youngson, Robert M. *The Surgery Book: An Illustrated Guide to 73 of the Most Common Operations.* New York: St. Martin's Press, 1993.

Web Sites

American Association of Health Plans. (August 15, 1997). AAHP Fact Sheets: Access Retrieved September 28, 1998 from the World Wide Web: *http://www.aahp.org/services/consumer_information/facts/access.html*

Bettinger, J. (January 9, 1994). Kaiser Permanente. *San Jose Mercury News.* Retrieved October 26, 1998 from the World Wide Web: *http://www.sjmercury.com/resources/search/search_archive.html.*

Heath Care Financing Administration. (1998). National Heath Care Expenditures: National health expenditures aggregate, per capita, percent distribution, and annual percentage change by source of funds: Calendar years 1960-96 [Data file posted on the World Wide Web]. Retrieved September 28, 1998 from the World Wide Web: *http://www.hcfa.gov/stats/nhe-oact/nhe.htm.*

Kaiser Permanente. (1998). About Kaiser Permanente - Who We Are. Retrieved October 26, 1998 from the World Wide Web: *http://www.kaiserpermanente.org/about/whoweare.html.*

National Committee for Quality Assurance. (September 23, 1998). State of Managed Care Quality Press Release [Press release posted on the World Wide Web]. Retrieved September 25, 1998 from the World Wide Web: *http://www.ncqa.org/news/sofmcrel.htm.*

Journals and Periodicals

Anders, George. "Money Machines: HMOs Pile up Billions in Costs, Try to Decide What to do With it." *Wall Street Journal,* December 21, 1994.

Badger, J. "Calming the Anxious Patient." *American Journal of Nursing,* 94 (5), (1994): 46-50.

Breemhaar, B., Van den Borne, H.W. "Effects of Education and Support for Surgical Patients: The Role of Perceived Control." *Patient Education and Counseling,* 18, (1991): 199-210.

Caldwell, L.N. "The Influence of Preference for Information on Preoperative Stress and Coping in Surgical Outpatients." *Applied Nursing Research.* 4 (4), (1991): 177-183.

Fromm, C.G., Metzler, D.J. "Preparing Your Older Patient for Surgery." *RN,* 56 (1), (1993): 38-42.

Greenberg, I., and M.L. Rodburg."The Role of Prepaid Group Practice in Relieving the Medical Care Crises." *Harvard Law Review.* 84. (1971): 887-1004.

Groah, L.K. "The Perioperative Role." *Operating Room Nursing,* Reston, VA.: Reston Publishing Co., 1983.

Horne, D., Vatanidis, P., and A. Careri. "Preparing Patients for Invasive Medical and Surgical Procedures I: Adding Behavioral and Cognitive Interventions." *Behavioral Medicine* 20: (1994): 5-26.

Jackson, M.F., "High Risk Surgical Patients," *Today's O.R. Nurse*, 19 (12), (1998): 26-33.

Kapp, M.B. "Elder Care: Informed, Assisted Delegated Consent for Elderly Patients." *AORN Journal* 52 (4), (1990): 857-862.

Larson, Eric. "The Soul of an HMO." *Time Magazine*, January 22, 1996.

Laufman H. "Environmental Concerns in Surgery in the 1990s." *Today's OR Nurse* 12 (10), (1990): 41-48, 50-51.

Luft, H.S., and R.H. Miller. "Patient Selection in a Competitive Health System." *Health Affairs* 7 (3), (1988): 97-119.

Patton, Rebecca. "What You Must Know Before you go to the Hospital." *Redbook* March 1996.

Palermo. B.J. "Capitation on Trial." *California Medicine* February 1996.

Spargins, Ellyn E. "Beware Your HMO." *Newsweek* October 23, 1995.

Wilensky, G.R. and L.F. Rossiter. "Patient Self Selection in HMOs." *Health Affairs* 5 (1), (1986): 66-80.